MW00995155

THE BIBLE STUDY FOR ADVANCE CARE PLANNING

I'll Have It
GOD'S
WAY

*Living Fully
Now and Into Your Forever*

TAKING CONTROL OF END-OF-LIFE DECISIONS

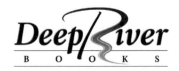

I'll Have It God's Way: Living Fully Now and Into Your Forever
Copyright @ 2018 by Hattie Bryant
Published by Deep River Books
Sisters, Oregon
www.deepriverbooks.com

Scripture marked NIV is taken from the Holy Bible, New International Version®, NIV® Copyright © 1973, 1978, 1984, 2011 by Biblica, Inc.® Used by permission. All rights reserved worldwide.

Scripture marked CEV is taken from the Contemporary English Version®. Copyright © 1995 by American Bible Society. Used by permission.

Scripture marked ERV is taken from the Easy-to-Read Version, Copyright © 2006 by Bible League international.

Scripture marked ESV is taken from The Holy Bible, English Standard Version. ESV® Text Edition: 2016. Copyright © 2001 by Crossway Bibles, a publishing ministry of Good News Publishers.

Scripture marked GNT is taken from the Good News Translation® (Today's English Version, Second Edition). Copyright © 1992 American Bible Society. All rights reserved.

Scripture marked GWT is taken from GOD'S WORD®, © 1995 God's Word to the Nations. Used by permission of Baker Publishing Group.

Scripture marked ICB is taken from The Holy Bible, International Children's Bible® Copyright© 1986, 1988, 1999, 2015 by Tommy Nelson™, a division of Thomas Nelson. Used by permission.

Scripture marked KJV is taken from The Holy Bible, King James Version. Public Domain.

Scripture marked TLB is taken from The Living Bible copyright © 1971 by Tyndale House Foundation. Used by permission of Tyndale House Publishers Inc., Carol Stream, Illinois 60188. All rights reserved.

Scripture marked MSG is taken from The Message. Copyright © 1993, 1994, 1995, 2000, 2001, 2002. Used by permission of NavPress Publishing Group.

Scripture marked NASB is taken from the New American Standard Bible. Copyright © 1960, 1962, 1963, 1968, 1971, 1972, 1973, 1975, 1977, 1995 by the Lockman Foundation. Used by permission.

Scripture marked NCV is taken from the New Century Version®. Copyright © 2005 by Thomas Nelson. Used by permission. All rights reserved.

Scripture marked NLT is taken from the Holy Bible, New Living Translation, copyright © 1996, 2004, 2015 by Tyndale House Foundation. Used by permission of Tyndale House Publishers, Inc., Carol Stream, Illinois 60188. All rights reserved.

Scripture marked TPT is taken from The Passion Translation®. Copyright © 2017 by BroadStreet Publishing® Group, LLC. Used by permission. All rights reserved. thePassionTranslation.com.

Scripture marked NET is taken from the NET Bible® Copyright ©1996–2006 by Biblical Studies Press, L.L.C. http://netbible.com All rights reserved.

Scripture marked ISV is taken from The Holy Bible: International Standard Version®. Copyright © 2003 by The ISV Foundation. Used by permission of Davidson Press, Inc. All rights reserved internationally.

Scripture marked PH is taken from the New Testament in Modern English by J. B. Phillips. Copyright © 1960, 1972 J. B. Phillips. Administered by The Archbishops' Council of the Church of England. Used by permission.

Scripture marked VOICE is taken from The Voice Bible. Copyright © 2012 Thomas Nelson, Inc. The Voice™ translation © 2012 Ecclesia Bible Society All rights reserved.

ISBN – 13: 9781632694935
LOC: 2018964950

Printed in the USA
2018—First Edition

26 25 24 23 22 21 20 19 18   10 9 8 7 6 5 4 3 2 1

Cover design by Robin Black, Inspirio Design

Contents

My Story 4

Mom's Story 5

What Happened to Me When I Turned 60 7

How to Use This Study 9

SESSION ONE 11

    Homework 17

    Reading 1: A Taste of Eden 23

    Reading 2: Seek God's Truth 31

SESSION TWO 49

    Homework 58

    Reading 3: There's a Gentle Path 65

SESSION THREE 77

    Homework 88

    Reading 4: Create a Circle of Care 95

SESSION FOUR 105

    Homework 110

SESSION FIVE 115

    Homework 119

    Reading 5: Start Living in God's Kingdom Now 121

SESSION SIX 129

    Homework 135

APPENDICES 139

My Directive in Essay Form 140

Cliff Notes for the Psalms. 143

My Gift to My Circle of Care 148

My Story

*For God so loved the world that he gave his one and only son that whoever
believes in him shall not perish but have eternal life.*
— JOHN 3:16, NIV

It was a Saturday night in 1958, I was eight years old, and my mom and dad decided it was time to understand what I had been learning in Sunday school, from the sermons on Sunday, and from our Bible reading done at the dinner table every night. They opened my own copy of the Bible, a small King James Version with a white leatherette cover, inscribed with John 3:16. I immediately recognized it as probably the most famous scripture of all time and I had already memorized it. When my parents asked me what it meant, in typical eight-year-old fashion with utter sincerity, I replied, "I guess it means what it says."

They pressed on. "You know, Hattie, this verse was written for you. The whole Bible was written for you. So we want to know if you believe this for yourself. Do you?" I nodded my head "yes." That night, I accepted Jesus Christ as my Savior and Lord and asked him to forgive me for my sins and asked him to lead me through the rest of this life.

The next day, my dad, who was an ordained Baptist minister, baptized me in the little old wooden church where we were members. Dressed in a simple white gown, I was submerged while in the arms of my earthly father, and came up out of the water imagining being lifted up by the arms of my heavenly Father. The older I get, the more powerful the image is: me going down under that water, the child my parents brought into this world, and coming up out of it as the child of the creator of the universe. My old biological life is dead. I am risen up, just as Jesus Christ rose up and walked out of his grave.

Hattie Bryant

Mom's Story

ANNABELLE BRYANT, 1915–1990

Precious in the sight of the Lord is the death of his saints.

— PSALM 116:15, KJV

It was October 9, 1990 when Dad called me to say that Mom had suffered a stroke and was in the hospital in New Orleans where my sister lived at the time. My brother and I lived in other states but promised to get there are soon as possible.

I learned quickly that when a person has a stroke, it becomes a waiting game for the family and medical staff, as everyone watches to see what aspects of the damaged functionality will return.

During Mom's six-week stay in the hospital, I made it a point to fly in about once a week and stayed as many days as I could before I had to fly out to my next job. In the fourth week, things got worse; she closed her eyes and didn't open them for days. The end of the fifth week of her hospitalization was Thanksgiving Day, November 22, and when I arrived, I noticed immediately that Mom's condition was very different. The first shock was her blank face. The second shock was the feeding tube that had been inserted because the doctors and nurses said she could no longer swallow; they were only doing what they thought was best, in the absence of any information to the contrary.

My eyes told me that watching and waiting would lead to no improvement, only deterioration. I also knew she and dad both had living wills and that hers stated that she did not want life-prolonging care if she became incapacitated—so why was this happening? Alone with my mom that Thanksgiving morning, I picked up the chart and found that she was being given something daily called desmopressin nasal (DDAVP nasal spray), a manmade form of a hormone that is produced naturally in the pituitary gland. This hormone is important for many functions including regulating how the body uses water.

It was comforting that Mom's primary care doctor was making rounds on Thanksgiving Day. I asked the doctor about the nasal spray and he explained that the endocrinologist (a specialist in the area of human metabolism, especially hormones) prescribed it. The stroke had severely damaged the part of her brain that created the hormone that tells the kidneys how to handle water, and so the nasal spray was telling her kidneys to keep a proper fluid balance.

I asked him whether Mom was going to get better. The doctor said no, this was as good as Mom was going to get, and that she would have to be moved to a nursing home as there was nothing more to be done for her at the hospital. Her condition was no longer acute but chronic, which meant that she could only live for a very long time with artificial feeding and the nasal spray.

One of the nurses caring for Mom had told us that without the nasal spray she thought it would take about one week for Mom to fully wind down out of this physical world. I told Mom's primary doctor that I knew she didn't want to be kept alive this way and asked him to stop the nasal spray immediately. He wisely calmed me down and suggested I speak with my father, sister, and brother.

When I told my father about the situation later that evening and asked about her living will, he confirmed that she had a living will, but that no one had asked for it. He thought that meant that the doctors believed Mom was going to get better because they kept treating her. With the misunderstanding explained, he agreed with me that we needed to let her go to her forever home.

That day, the social worker for my mom's case came to the room and wanted to meet me. She took me out into the hall and said, "Everybody needs a Hattie." She is the reason for this book. *Finally, I have written the book that the social worker said everybody needs.*

God's Lessons for Me While Watching My Mom Die

1. I learned that living wills cannot be honored unless the doctors have seen them. Even though my parents had planned ahead and had prepared living wills, like so many other Americans, those documents were in a safe place somewhere. Some folks are known to put these healthcare instructions with the wills they have created to tell family and friends who is going to get grandfather's watch and other assets.

2. We cannot expect doctors or nurses to read our minds and know which and how much treatment we want to receive. This is especially true in a medical world defined more and more by specialty, where treatment is often parsed out among several doctors with various areas of expertise and often without communication with other treating physicians or family before administering care. In Mom's case, the endocrinologist thought he was doing the right thing and prescribing something beneficial for my mom. Or, maybe he was simply doing what his training and conscience told him to do, without knowing her or her history or what her wishes or the wishes of our family were in this situation.

3. One of the benefits of modern medicine is that there are other healthcare specialists who are involved in the patient's care, *in addition to* the physician specialists. Just like the social worker who comforted me, we too can have that level of understanding and support in our time of need—if only we know to ask.

Hattie Bryant

What Happened to Me
When I Turned 60

I n 2010 I turned sixty and I remember saying to myself, "I have lived more years than I have left. Who is going to do for me what I did for my mom? Who will ask the hard questions? Why did the doctors do what they did and why do they keep doing what they do? What's the difference between medical well-being and physical well-being? *Finally, what, if anything, does my belief in Jesus Christ have to do with the choices I make while I am still healthy and when my health fails?"*

Finding the answers to these questions for myself led me to national meetings of physicians, nurses, and social workers. It led me back to school, where I studied in the University of Southern California graduate program in Gerontology. After five years of study and at the counsel of physicians and nurses who mentored me, I wrote the faith-neutral book *I'll Have It My Way,* so that it could be used in their offices and hospitals. I subsequently produced a lecture based on *I'll Have It My Way* that airs on public television stations. I am grateful that today, thousands of copies are out there guiding individuals and their families to think about the important choices they need to make about their health and care while they are healthy.

However, from the beginning, God's call on my heart was to write a book for those believers of John 3:16, "that whosoever believes in him shall not perish but have eternal life." So, when I learned from my "research" that Christians die just like everyone else, I was shocked. I had a front row seat at my mom's death and confirmed that not even Christians are good at facing death. My own father, an ordained Baptist minister with a master's degree in theology, was incapable of dealing with doctors due to his grief.

I learned I could not—nor was it right to—depend on loved ones to follow through on my wishes. Moreover, I could not expect any healthcare professional to read my mind. It is my job to think ahead and figure out how to prevent many of the things that have become standard care at end-of-life (for example, breathing and feeding tubes) from being done to me.

My healthcare directive is the result of twenty-five years of thinking about how I would like to see the last few years of my life play out.

This thinking has all been done while watching the forward march of medicine and its full unquestioning embrace by Christians. My research for *I'll Have It My Way* taught me that pursuing God's goals for me might require me to swim upstream, against the heavy tide of much of what modern medicine has to offer.

Just because everyone else allows medicine to do anything to them doesn't mean I have to. I now understand why I felt overwhelmed with grief to see my mom dying on Thanksgiving Day of 1990 and why I—a very strong, healthy accomplished forty-year old—was diminished to a feeling of helplessness.

I now know that a sweet, peaceful death will not come out of the natural flow of our lives in this twenty-first century.

I now know that most of modern medicine focuses on our physical well-being, and so we must step up to partner with our Creator to take charge of our total well-being. And, we all are going to have to do these five things:

1. Accept That We Are Not God and We Will All Die
2. Learn the Limits of Modern Medicine
3. Understand Our Healthcare Choices
4. Choose a Proxy and Provide Specific Instructions
5. Start Living in God's Kingdom Now

While 70 percent of Americans say they want to die at home surrounded by friends and family, more than 70 percent are dying in institutions and many are dying alone. By 2020, 40 percent of Americans who die will be alone and in an institution.[1] The learning, thinking, praying, writing, and sharing you do in these pages will give you a very good chance of having the kind of peaceful death you expect to have as the chosen child of God that you are.

---

1   *The Economist, April 29, 2017, accessed November 26, 2018, https://www.economist.com/international/2017/04/29/a-better-way-to-care-for-the-dying

How to Use This Study

Welcome to *I'll Have It God's Way*. You're here, and I am already giving you a standing ovation! Most people live in denial or fear of this topic and want to pretend it is something that happens to other people. Simply by holding this book in your hand, you have taken a step most won't take. Augustine wrote, "The happy life is joy based on the truth."[2] It follows then that unhappiness stems from not liking the truth and rejecting it, as it makes us uneasy. You are entering into uneasy territory, but don't worry. This guide was created to make the difficult doable. Everything you need to create the only advance care directive you need for yourself or loved ones is right here. This will be more detailed than what you might have done in the past and it will allow you to take control of end-of-life care. If your goal is to live fully now and into your forever, I will show you what you can do now to make this dream come true.

Are you ready to talk and think about what nobody wants to talk and think about? OK, let's get started.

Use with a Group or Not
I'll Have It God's Way is for anyone over 65, for the adult children of the elderly, and for the family caregivers of the seriously ill or frail. Adult children and family caregivers will participate in the study and then bring what they learned to those they are caring for. This becomes a communication tool for them to get the sick and frail to think, talk, and write. It is designed to be used with your small group, or you can use it by yourself, or perhaps with all of your family. I want it to be easy and flexible, which is why the videos are posted for free and unlimited use on YouTube.

What You Need
- This book.
- A Bible.
- Access to the videos, available on DVD or for free online. The free videos can be accessed at www.illhaveitgodsway.com/biblestudy.

Timing
My hope is that you by yourself or you in your group can walk through this study in six one-hour sessions, with some reading and writing homework assignments you will need to do on your own schedule. While a typical study group might meet weekly, there is always room for adaption. Frankly, if you are in a hurry, you could do this study in a weekend or simply find a schedule that works for you.

Between the Sessions
There's too much to learn, process, and personalize in the six one-hour sessions, so I have given you things to do on your own before you move ahead. Do the assignments in small bites or in one sitting. Make it work for you.

The Group Leader
The leader can start the videos, keep track of time or choose a timekeeper, read questions out loud, and encourage everyone in the group to participate. Each person's shared experience and thoughts will add depth that could bring more insight than any one reading or any one video contained here. If you're doing this alone, then you are the leader.

---

2   Saint Augustine, *Confessions* (Oxford: Oxford University Press, 1991), 199.

Accept That We Are Not God and We Will All Die

Big Word for This Session: TRUTH

And you will know the truth, and the truth will set you free.
— JOHN 8:32, TLB

Opening

Optional Listening: "I Can Only Imagine" at the link found on this page: illhaveitgodsway.com/biblestudy

Opening Prayer: Father God, show us fresh insight now, as we open ourselves to you. We ask this humbly in the name of Jesus, Amen.

Play the Session One video.

Available on the DVD or from the link found on this page: illhaveitgodsway.com/biblestudy

Video Discussion:

1. What surprised Hattie about her mom's death?

2. How does denying our reality affect us?

3. Do you know some elders who are not elders? How would you describe the way they live their lives?

4. What can we do to grow wise, loving, and free from the fear of death?

As Christians, we want to reject what our secular culture calls death—and reframe this to mean, for us, a leaving or our escape from the confines of physicality. Jesus made it perfectly clear that those of us who put our confidence in him will not "taste" death.

Going Deeper

5. Read aloud John 11:26. What promise does this make?

6. Read aloud Romans 8:18. What promise does this make?

7. Why is it so hard for us to even talk about death?

8. Do we tend to fear the unknown in general, and the afterlife in particular? Could we have this fear—fear is the root of denial—because we haven't thought about death enough to form our own belief about it?

9. What experiences have you had watching people die? Were they spiritually mature and found it easy to accept their situation, or did they struggle with denial/fear? What were you thinking as you watched this person? What will you want to do differently? What will you want to emulate?

Play the video clip from FAQs: Is Death Painful?
Available on the DVD or from the link found on this page:
illhaveitgodsway.com/biblestudy

10. Why would a dying woman say, "Dying doesn't cause suffering; resistance to dying causes suffering"?

"But me? God snatches me from the clutch of death, he reaches down and grabs me. . . . We aren't immortal. We don't last long. Like our dogs, we age and weaken. And die."

— Psalm 49:15, 20, MSG

11. Are you ready to let go and let God have your mind, body, and soul? If not, why not? Places to go? People to see? Things to do? Things to learn?

12. Modern medicine has tools for our physical pain, but it can't help with our spiritual pain. What can you do now to get spiritually ready to relax into your eternal spirit?

13. Read the description of the Kübler-Ross Model and accompanying verses on the next page and answer the following questions.

    a. Do these psalms comfort you and help you feel connected to the ancient faithful? If they struggled, then do we all? Will you?

    b. Why will it be hard for us to skip through Kübler-Ross's first four stages of death—denial, anger, bargaining, depression? What would our acceptance that death is coming look like to others?

    c. Can you imagine that it will be easier for you to accept the fact that you are dying when that time comes than it will be for your family to accept the fact that you are dying? Why or why not?

In his sermon "When You're Hoping for a Miracle," Rick Warren refers to Elisabeth Kübler-Ross to describe how spiritually unprepared people react to a difficult diagnosis. Read them together, then discuss the questions afterward:

Denial (a form of fear) = This is not happening to me!

"I am frightened inside; the terror of death has attacked me" (Psalm 55:4, NCV).

Anger = Why is this happening to me?

"I was overcome with [anger]. The more I thought, the more troubled I became; I could not keep from asking: 'LORD, how long will I live? When will I die? Tell me how soon my life will end'" (Psalm 39:3–4, GNB).

Bargaining = I promise to ... if you'll let me live.

"You can never pay God enough to stay alive forever and be safe from death" (Psalm 49:8–9, CEV).

Depression = I just don't care anymore.

"I'm at the end of my rope, my life in ruins. I'm fading away to nothing, passing away" (Psalm 109:22–23, MSG).

Acceptance = I'm ready for whatever happens.

"I am trusting you, O LORD, saying, 'You are my God!' My future is in your hands" (Psalm 31:14–15, NLT).

Closing Prayer:

Father, help us see what you want us to see. Dispel any fears or anxieties we have about our own death and the deaths of those we love. Set us free! In Christ's name we ask, Amen.

Before the next group session, complete the following homework and Readings 1 and 2. The first reading goes deeper into the topics covered in this session, while the second will prepare you for discussion in Session Two. Don't worry; this is the only time I'll ask you to do this much reading between sessions.

HOMEWORK

Looking at Yourself

1. Read the following statements and check the answer that most agrees with your thinking. There is no right or wrong answer.

	TRUE	FALSE
I'm afraid of the dying process		
I'm afraid to die		
Others depend upon me		
Others depend upon my financial resources		
I'm afraid my spouse will fall apart without me		
I can't afford to die		
I'm afraid of a long, slow decline		
I'm afraid my children will fight over my assets		
I'm not sure of my salvation		
I'm not sure of the resurrection		
I'm not sure there's a heaven		
I don't want to be a burden on my family		
I don't want to lose my independence		
I have financial obligations I don't want to leave to others		
I don't want to be in pain		
I haven't done all that I dreamed I would do with my life		
I've made mistakes I'd like to fix		
I have regrets		

Any statement that you marked TRUE reveals a concern that will keep you in denial. This is not where God wants you to be.

2. Prioritize the worries you marked "True" by numbering them in order of how you should work to resolve them.

3. Make a list of steps you can take to work on each of those worries.

4. Some of your worries are due to what Fritz Perls called "unfinished business." **To take care of unfinished business, make a list** here of people you need to talk with. These are people to whom you may need to say, "I'm sorry," "Thank you," or "I love you."

This will not be easy, but you're not alone. Remember, you carry inside of you the Holy Spirit who was put in you by God himself (1 Corinthians 3:16). Have a look at my translation of Colossians 1:22: *You are a temple of God and the Spirit of God dwells in you.*

> By dying for you, Christ brought you over to God's side and put your life together whole and holy in his sight and free from blemish and free from accusation.

5. What does this verse mean to you? How does this encourage you to face fears, especially the fear of death?

Hattie Bryant

Put Your Forever With God Top of Mind

6. How much do you think about your forever in your new and glorified body in the new heaven and new earth? If not at all, why not?

7. What does the Bible tell us about our future with God? Look up these verses, and write what you learn from them about your life after this life.

Luke 23:43 *... today you will be with me in Paradise*

Psalm 23 *We'll go through the valley not stay - He will be with me - goodness & mercy will follow me all the days of my life*

John 14:2-3 *my Father has many dwelling places. He will come again for me and take me to the place He has made for me. He will receive me and I will be with Him always!*

Isaiah 65:17 *For behold, I create new heavens and a new earth, and the former things shall not be remembered or come to mind.*

Colossians 3:1-3 *Set your mind on things above - not on things on the earth - For you died and your life is hidden w/ Christ in God. When Christ who is our life appears, then you will also appear w/ Him in glory*

2 Corinthians 4:8 *We are afflicted in every way, but not crushed; perplexed, but not driven to despair*

Revelation 21:1-3 *Behold, the dwelling place of God is with man. He will dwell with them, and They will be His people, and God himself will be with them as their God.*

8. How can you keep your eye cast to eternity when there's so much to do here? Even Paul had tension over this dilemma. Look up Philippians 1:21 (NIV), and fill in the blanks:

For to me, to live is __**Christ**__ *and to die is* __**gain**__ *. If I am to go on living in the body, this will mean fruitful labor for me. Yet what shall I choose? I do not know!*

Does this tell us that Paul is leaving the choice to God? Explain.

In 2 Corinthians 5:6, 8 (NASB), we learn more about Paul: "knowing that while we are at home in the body we are absent from the Lord . . . we . . . prefer rather to be absent from the body and to be at home with the Lord."

9. Read Hebrews 11:13–16. What did so many men and women of faith have in common?

10. How do we grow our faith?

11. What will more faith in God do for our outlook on life and death?

---

12. Now, reach back to David. Read Psalm 42:1–2.

 a. What is David asking for in this passage?

 b. Describe David's emotions.

Yearning for the renewal of all things and for the return of Christ helps us prioritize our time here, it takes us out of the driver's seat and puts God there where he belongs, and it reminds us that this is a temporary place where we are only being prepared for eternity with God.

Hattie Bryant

13. Imagine you have been given a difficult diagnosis. Remember on page 18, where I mentioned tying up loose ends? Write love letters and thank-you notes to the people listed there. Here's one I wrote to my husband:

Dear Bruce,

You, my darling, are my one and only. What a gift God gave to me when he put you in my life. What fun it is to live with the bravest person I know. What joy it is to live with a man who is seeking after the heart of God. How freeing it is to live with a man who knows no fear. How comforting it is to live with a man who tells me that he loves and adores me. How invigorating to live with a man who never wants to go down the same road twice. What an adventure you are.

When you wrap your arms around me, I feel safe. When you call to me, I feel wanted. When you eat my cooking, I feel appreciated. I can't imagine earthbound life without you.

I love you with all my heart.

Hattie

Here's one to a girlfriend:

Dear RWG,

Who would have ever dreamed that when we sat outside a mutual friend's home where we met for the first time that our friendship would come to this! I have had many wonderful women in my life over the years but no one has taught me more about friendship than you. Even though you're MUCH younger than me, I want to be like you when I grow up. And even though you have many, many friends, you make me feel like your favorite and I know that is not true. Thank you for loving me, for encouraging me, for flying all over the country and running through airports with me. Thank you for praying for me and for being THE Proverbs 31 woman that you are.

Hattie

Books you can read to strengthen your belief in heaven:

Heaven, by Randy Alcorn

A Place Called Heaven, by Robert Jeffress

Surprised by Hope, by N. T. Wright

A New Heaven and a New Earth, by J. Richard Middleton

God Dwells Among Us: Expanding Eden to the Ends of the Earth,
    by G. K. Beale and Mitchell Kim

All Things New, by John Eldredge

Verse for meditation:

Philippians 1:21 (NIV): For to me, to live is Christ and to die is gain.

Before the next session, be sure to complete Readings 1 and 2 on pages 23–48. You can also review the Session One videos at illhaveitgodsway.com/biblestudy.

A Taste of Eden

Accept That We Are Not God and We Will All Die
Learn the Limits of Modern Medicine
Understand Our Healthcare Choices
Choose a Proxy and Provide Specific Instructions
Start Living in God's Kingdom Now

The life of mortals is like grass, they flourish like a flower of the field;
the wind blows over it and it is gone.
— PSALM 103:15–16, NIV

Is death optional? Of course not, but our behavior looks like we think this. Our wealthy American culture, soaked in confidence that we can do anything and achieve anything, has us all caught up in a web of secular deception about death and dying. Sadly, this same deception has many of today's Christians ensnared in its tangled web as well. It's far easier to be conformed to the ways of the world, and far more difficult to think about death and talk about death with ease and confidence as a believer in Christ.

As Christians we must think about and talk about death, not in the terms of the secular world, but because it is the joyful way we experience what we say we believe. The Bible is clear: We will not experience death—at least as the secular world thinks of it. Yes, our body will break down and quit, but as the Bible teaches us, we are not our body. We are more than flesh. Christ conquered death so this should not be a problem for us, but it is. When death comes to us, most of us will say to God, "I'm not ready yet." It is the ultimate test of our belief in God's promise, and on the question of how much we really believe, our actions fail us.

Elisabeth Kübler-Ross was a physician who became famous by studying the dying. Her 1969 book *On Death and Dying* is considered by many to be the "bible" on the topic by modern medicine. She determined there were five stages in the dying process: denial, anger, bargaining, depression, and acceptance. While modern medicine and even personal experience with those who have died may lead us to believe this is how dying is done, there is no reason it has to be so for believers in Christ. We know where we came from, we know where we're going; so as Christians, we can stay focused on our glorious truth that we will never die. Our bodies will fail us, but our spirits never stop, never quit, and never wander.

Paradise Lost . . . and Found

God never intended for us to die. His dream for us was to live with him in paradise from day one and never get off that path. The day that Adam and Eve were arrogant enough to play God was the day our trouble with death started. Genesis 2:17 (MSG) says, "God commanded the Man, 'You can eat from any tree in the garden, except from the Tree-of-Knowledge-of-Good-and-Evil. Don't eat from it. The moment you eat from that tree, you're dead.'" Metaphorically, death came to our spirits, and physically we were given lives that would now include suffering, sickness, and eventually death. Adam and Eve made the choice, and we inherited the results.

In a sermon called "A Path through Suffering," delivered on January 6, 2008, pastor and writer Tim Keller says, "When God made the world he didn't make disease in it. It wasn't a place of death. Disease, disaster, and death are not things God actually made. They are forces of darkness that were unleashed when we turned away from God. When we rebelled against God, the fabric of this world began to unravel. We unleashed these forces."[3]

John Eldredge writes, "Death is such an assault on the soul. . . . Death is so hostile, so explosive to God's design for us, the soul experiences it as trauma. . . . Our souls were never meant to go through this, so we reel like a ship in high seas."[4]

Bound by Religion

Describing death as Keller and Eldredge do, as "forces of darkness," "hostile," "explosive," and a "trauma," we may not be surprised by the findings of Herman Feifel in his 1959 book *The Meaning of Death.*[5] He found that religious persons are more afraid to die than the nonreligious; and new research confirms that those who say that they are Christians are just as afraid to die as others, and are just as afraid to let loved ones die as are the nonreligious.

In his sermon preached on May 14, 2011, "You Will Never See Death!" pastor and author John Piper says that the writer of Hebrews, "believes that all human beings are enslaved their whole life by the fear of death even when they don't know it."[6] We can read for ourselves Hebrews 2:14 (MSG), where it says, "Since the children are made of flesh and blood, it's logical that the Savior took on flesh and blood in order to rescue them by his death. By embracing death, taking it into himself, he destroyed the Devil's hold on death and freed all who cower through life, scared to death of death."

---

3   Tim Keller, "A Path through Suffering," January 6, 2008, accessed July 4, 2018, https://player.fm/series/timothy-keller-sermons-podcast-by-gospel-in-life-83408/questions-of-suffering.

4   John Eldredge, "We Live Forever," Ransomed Heart, August 22, 2016, accessed November 1, 2017, https://ransomedheart.com/blogs/john/we-live-forever.

5   Herman Feifel, *The Meaning of Death* (New York: McGraw-Hill, 1959), 121.

6   John Piper, "You Will Never See Death!" May 14, 2011, accessed July 4, 2018, https://www.desiringgod.org/messages/you-will-never-see-death.

In the same sermon, Piper calls us out and says (emphasis added), "Fear of death produces a pervasive, lifelong bondage—even when we don't realize it, fear is haunting our choices, making us cautious, wary, restrained, confined, narrow, tight, robbing us of risk and adventure and dreams for the sake of Christ and his kingdom and the cause of love in the world. Why do you live such cautious lives? Why do you devote so much energy to security? Without our even knowing it, *fear of death is a slave master binding us with invisible ropes, confining us to small, safe, innocuous, self-centered lives.* Jesus sets us free!"

Even as we read God's Word and hear his promises preached, we come face to face with the reality of our unbelief. On some level of our consciousness, we continue to wonder if we are going to heaven or hell. Out of that insecurity comes the reflexive but futile mindset that if only we work harder, become more pious, throw a few more dollars in the offering plate we can still earn—or buy—our way to our forever home. The reality is just the opposite. To grasp all of what Jesus came to do, we can start killing off the religion in our lives to make room for the only one we need to live fully, boldly, fearlessly all the way into heaven.

The gospel is not about religion it is about relation. It is about the finite-to-infinite connection to our Creator granted to us through the infusion of the spirit put in us by God himself. Dallas Willard says we are, "never-ceasing spiritual beings with a unique eternal destiny to count for good in God's great universe."[7] How can we live out our eternal destiny if we hold on to these flawed and broken bodies? When you are told that our life in this familiar place is fragile and frail, think of your life with God as the grand new beginning for which you want to do your utmost to prepare.

Paul, who some would say was the greatest Christian to ever live, teaches us to laugh in the face of death. He wrote in 1 Corinthians 15:55 (GWT), "Death, where is your victory? Death, where is your sting?" Just ahead of that, Paul says that our flesh and blood will not make it to heaven. That tells me, if I am going to get to see Jesus face to face, I have to let go of this body and believe, as Paul also said, "For to me, living means living for Christ, and dying is even better" (Philippians 1:21, NLT).

Too Good to Believe

As Christians, we know the plan God put in place. It stands to reason that if we think and plan ahead, we can take the assurance of God's plan to the grave and shake the fear of death that grips most others. Haven't we all heard and read, "The truth sets you free," and "Perfect love casts out all fear"? They sound nice, but for some reason we have a hard time internalizing them and applying them when things in our life go beyond our control.

---

7   Dallas Willard, *The Divine Conspiracy: Recovering Our Hidden Life* (New York: HarperCollins, 1997), 21.

My own experience may shed some light. From childhood on, I have spent my life trying very hard to be good, to work hard, always striving to be responsible and self-sufficient. I was proud of my independence, and it took me a long time (and a time-out by God) to realize that independence had also made me question how much I really needed God. My life was going smoothly, and I was always able to get up each morning and make things happen—or at least *think* I was the one making things happen. Now I know I can't even breathe for myself.

It took God putting me in time-out for nearly ten years before I began to get the glory of the story. It is all too good to be true, right?

- Jesus really died for me? (Isaiah 53:5; Romans 5:8)
- Jesus really loves me? (John 15:12–13; 2 Corinthians 5:21)
- Jesus really wants me as his friend? (John 15:15)
- Jesus is ready, willing and able to give me everything I need if I just ask? (John 15:16)
- Jesus is in me, with me and for me? (Colossians 1:27)
- My name is tattooed on the palm of God's hand? (Isaiah 49:16)
- He knows the number of hairs on my head, and even as I lose hair everyday he is actually counting and cares about the number? (Luke 12:7)
- He knows my heart is broken over mistakes I have made, and he still wants me with him forever? (Isaiah 43:25)
- He follows my coming and going and will never leave me? (Psalm 139)
- He is knocking on my front door and wants to come and eat with me and enjoy a two-way conversation—and I don't have to work myself into a frenzy like Martha before he shows up? (Revelation 3:20)

Writing to the church in Rome, Paul said, "But God demonstrated his own love for us in this: While we were still sinners, Christ died for us" (Romans 5:8, NIV). *Us* means Christ died for you and Christ died for me. This means you and I deserve to die but Jesus took our place. "For God took the sinless Christ and poured into him our sins. Then, in exchange, he poured God's goodness into us!" (2 Corinthians 5:21, TLB). Tim Keller explains this hard-to-believe truth when he says, "The irony of the gospel is that the only way to be worthy of it is to admit that you're completely unworthy of it."[8]

"But now he has reconciled you by his physical body through death to present you holy, without blemish, and blameless before him" (Colossians 1:22, NET). Take a moment to reflect on that verse. Why let fear take your joy, your peace, and your confidence in what God has already done?

---

8   Tim Keller, Twitter post, June 13, 2014, https://twitter.com/timkellernyc.

Hattie Bryant

Like me, you still may struggle with the idea that God would care about you when you don't deserve it. We're taught that God cares about the poor, the vulnerable, and the hungry, but by the world's standards we are not poor or vulnerable or hungry. He's provided far more than we need, so it's easy for us to forget how much we need him. If trusting God with mind, body, and soul is hard for you too, we can take comfort knowing that this is the struggle of the ages, and learn from those who go before us.

With a Song in Our Heart

Think of how hard life has been for humans since Adam and Eve's disobedience in the Garden of Eden. In our own country's short history, we can see in its founding and growth that the gospel, with the resurrection as its denouement pointing us to heaven, provided comfort to so many of the bold and the brave bound into slavery. Look what humans did with lives of misery when they had the resurrection in their hearts. When they embraced the promise of eternal life in a free and perfect place, the spirit of God in them inspired the melodies, rhythms, and lyrics. What these brothers and sisters in Christ gave to me, and to all of the Christians of the world, is treasure spun in the fire of life in a hard, mean world.

The Library of Congress has evidence that there were about six thousand spirituals composed by slaves and many refer to a better time, a better place, and a better life that will come when we leave these tired bones behind. These songs continue to live on because they spoke—and continue to speak—to the less-than-perfect life we may have on earth, even as we long for the day when all will be made perfect in his presence.[9]

Heaven was a recurring them in the songs of American slaves:

> Deep river, my home is over Jordan
> I'm bound for Canaan Land
> Swing low, sweet chariot
> De ol' ark's a-moverin and I' going home
> Blow your trumpet, Gabriel, blow me home to the new Jerusalem
> We are pilgrims here below and soon to glory we will go
> One of these mornings bright and fair, I want to cross over to see my Lord.
> Going to take my wings and fly the air, I want to cross over to see my Lord.

---

9   J. Richard Middleton says in his book, *A New Heaven and a New Earth*, that we are singing lies in church. While these old songs are comforting to those of us who grew up in church, he insists they limit our thinking about what God has for our future. I agree that the word "heaven" is simply too small to describe the glory we're headed into! Keep singing and imagine "heaven" is our entire cosmos redeemed and restored.

The theme of heaven was also found in the hymnody of the Puritans and those who settled our frontier. One of these songs, written in 1829, pops in my own head often.

We'll Work Till Jesus Comes

O land of rest, for thee I sigh!
When will the moment come when I shall lay my armor by and dwell in peace
   at home?

No tranquil joys on earth I know, No peaceful, shelt'ring dome;
This world's a wilderness of woe, This world is not my home.

To Jesus Christ I fled for rest; He bade me case to roam,
And lean for comfort on His breast till he conduct me home.

I sought at once my Savior's side; no more my steps shall roam;
With Him I'll brave death's chilling tide and reach my heav'nly home.

We'll work till Jesus comes, we'll work till Jesus comes,
We'll work till Jesus comes, and we'll be gathered home.

These songs endure because they continue to express the emotions felt by Christians across the ages.

Faith: "I am bound for the Promised Land, I am bound for the Promised Land. Oh, who will come and go with me? I am bound for the Promised Land."

Joy: "When we all get to heaven, what a day of rejoicing that will be. When we all see Jesus, we'll sing and shout the victory."

Comfort: "Jesus lover of my soul, let me to your bosom fly," a familiar song I imagined my mom sang when she knew her body was failing her, and one I sang at her funeral, "Some glad morning when this life is over, I'll fly away to a home far beyond the starry sky, I'll fly away."

Peace: "Steal Away," the song I sang at her graveside service:

Steal away, steal away, steal away to Jesus.
Steal away, steal away steal away home. I ain't got long to stay here.
My Lord he calls me, he calls me by the thunder.
The trumpet sounds within my heart. I ain't got long to stay here.

Hattie Bryant

Yearning for the renewal of all things and for the return of Christ helps us prioritize our time here. It takes us out of the driver's seat and puts God there where he belongs, and it reminds us that this is a temporary place where we are only being prepared for eternity with God, or as the words of this hymn reminds us: "This world is not my home. I'm just a passing through."

Letting go of this life is our only way to look into the face of Christ and hear him say, "Well done."

> We spring up like wildflowers in the desert and then wilt,
> transient as the shadow of a cloud.
> — Job 14:2, MSG

> A person's days are numbered; you have decreed the number of
> his months and have set limits he cannot exceed.
> — Job 14:5, NIV

> Teach us to number our days and recognize how few they are;
> help us to spend them as we should.
> — Psalm 90:12, TLB

> I have set before you life and death, blessings and curses.
> Now choose life, so that you and your children may live.
> — Deuteronomy 30:19, NIV

> Though our bodies are dying, our inner strength
> in the Lord is growing every day.
> — 2 Corinthians 4:16, TLB

Seek God's Truth

Accept That We Are Not God and We Will All Die

Learn the Limits of Modern Medicine

Understand Our Healthcare Choices

Choose a Proxy and Provide Specific Instructions

Start Living in God's Kingdom Now

How do you know what your life will be like tomorrow?

Your life is like the morning fog—it's here a little while, then it's gone.

— JAMES 4:14, NLT

A curse is placed on those who trust other people,

who depend on humans for strength,

who have stopped trusting the LORD.

— JEREMIAH 17:5, NCV

Cursed is the one who trusts in human strength and the abilities of mere mortals.

His very heart strays from the Eternal.

— JEREMIAH 17:5, VOICE

I, the LORD, have put a curse on those who turn from me

and trust in human strength.

— JEREMIAH 17:5, CEV

Modern medicine is fabulous until it isn't any more. It does have its ends, but most of us refuse to believe this. We have seen so much advancement in our lifetime that it's hard for us to imagine there is any medical problem that can't be solved. We simply need to get to the right place and find the right doctor, and we'll be cured to go back to what we were doing before we got sick.

None of us know the answer to the *when, where,* and *how* questions, but we all know with a 100 percent certainty that we are going to die. Isaac knew he didn't know when his death would come. He told his son Esau, "I am now an old man and don't know the day of my death" (Genesis 27:2, NIV). We'll talk more about this in session 4, but just note that Isaac was not in denial; he was putting plans in place for a future without his presence as the head of his household.

If we live, we die; that's the rule and God has stuck to the rule he put in place except for two men, Enoch and Elijah. They were so faithful, so after God's heart, that God saved them from the physical death process that even Jesus had to endure (Genesis 5:21-24; 2 Kings 2:11). Today, we are unlikely to see such miracles in our lifetime, and the reality of death coming to us all is reflected in a mathematical formula known as the Gompertz Law of Mortality. Simply stated, the older we become, the greater our chance of death—or as C. S. Lewis wrote in *A Grief Observed*, "Time itself is one more name for death."[10]

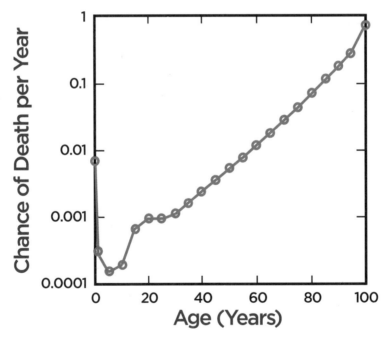

"When Christianity came into the world, pessimism was its main rival; today it is optimism" writes professor Peter Kreeft.[11] He goes on to say, "The essential difference

---

10 C. S. Lewis, *A Grief Observed* (New York: HarperCollins, 1961), 37.
11 Peter Kreeft, *I Burned for Your Peace: Augustine's Confessions Unpacked* (San Francisco: Ignatius Press, 2016), 2.

Hattie Bryant

between the medieval mind and the modern mind is right here. We spend most of our time and love and energy and perfection on science, which is the more perfect knowledge of less perfect things; while the medieval spent most of their time and love and energy on theology, which is the less perfect knowledge of the most perfect thing. The medieval mind was primitive in its science but profound in its theology. The modern mind is the reverse."[12]

We began the tossing out of our faith *in faith* in the late 1600s, when Isaac Newton invented calculus and then took his newfound notions of infinity and applied them to space and time. As an absolute frame of reference, science would soon discover that it no longer needed God to make things work. About one hundred years later, the theologians lost rank to the scientists, and today we seem to give science all the credit for giving us air conditioning, hair color, and cell phones.

While science takes center stage in our culture, Christians understand that every invention, every beautiful piece of music, every marvelous painting—all come from God. It doesn't matter about the heart of the human who invented penicillin. It doesn't matter that Richard Strauss and Pablo Picasso were atheists. God uses the gifts he gives to us, whether we recognize him or not. We can trust that the good done by modern medicine comes from God. There's no separating science and God, since God is science.

We Worship Little "g" Gods

Dr. Kreeft and other philosophers and theologians argue that we live in a post-Christian culture. No wonder Dr. Shannon Brownlee wrote in *Overtreated: Why Too Much Medicine Is Making Us Sicker and Poorer,* "Hospitals have been called the modern equivalent of Renaissance cathedrals."[13] Dr. Elisabeth Rosenthal described one major hospital system where she went to present a lecture as "a gleaming temple of healthcare."[14] Is this where we go to worship our one true evidence-based religion? Is Dr. Richard Della Penna right when he says that physicians tease that MD stands for Medical Deity?

> An astonishing 40% of Americans believe that medical technology can always save their lives. The old joke that Americans believe death is just one more disease to be cured is no longer a joke. No wonder Brookings Institution economist Henry Aaron—who has prominently called attention to all the problems of technology—has nonetheless written that any effort

---

12 Ibid, 177–118.

13 Shannon Brownlee, *Overtreated: Why Too Much Medicine Is Making Us Sicker and Poorer* (New York: Bloomsbury, 2007), 79.

14 Elisabeth Rosenthal, *An American Sickness: How Healthcare Became Big Business and How You Can Take It Back* (New York: Penguin, 2017), 48.

to curb the introduction of new technologies "beyond what is required for safety and efficacy would be sheer madness."[15]

We have become secularized to such an extent that we don't recognize that we have removed God and put science and medicine on the altar of our worship, and have put our health and faith in a pseudo-religion that is science-based, agnostic, and replete with its very own deity, the physician.

Maybe we think today's doctors are little "g" gods. Part wizard, part alchemist, they approach every illness with the years of education, the latest technologies and pharmaceuticals, and the self-confidence that numb our minds and mute our tongues from asking the questions we need to ask. So confident are we in their abilities that we refuse to see them for what they are: professionals who refuse to let us die because it will hurt their performance record or damage their ego, even when they know that there is nothing more they can do that will change the outcome of our illness.

Man Is Like a Breath

My mentor on my book *I'll Have It My Way*, Dr. Jack McNulty, started practicing medicine in 1951. He told me during one of my many interviews with him:

> The first successful use of cardiopulmonary resuscitation (CPR) was a watershed moment in medicine. This changed everything. I was there. I watched as the public was swept up. The public's reaction to CPR was misunderstood. In 1969 the media spread the word that a man who was dead was "brought back to life." This made the news and the public went crazy and started demanding CPR. There was a euphoria that overtook the country. People started believing that death is optional.

My friend Dr. Pat Gary is a third-generation physician. Although her father never said it out loud to her, Pat knew that he would turn and walk the other way when he heard "Code Blue" in the hospital where he practiced medicine for five decades. Pat got the sense that her father thought there was something very wrong with CPR, and that he would not have any part of it. Perhaps that is because he realized the truth of Psalm 144:4 (ESV):

> *Man is like a breath;*
> *his days are like a passing shadow.*

---

15 Daniel Callahan, "Health Care Costs and Medical Technology," in *From Birth to Death and Bench to Clinic: The Hastings Center Bioethics Briefing Book for Journalists, Policymakers, and Campaigns*, ed. Mary Crowley (Garrison, NY: The Hastings Center, 2008), 79–82.

Young doctors are writing now about the tragedy that CPR inflicts. An anesthesiologist in a large hospital, Dr. Margaret Overton, writes that only 5 percent of patients receiving hospital-based CPR are survivors who actually leave the hospital.

> We live in a society where we act first and think later, or don't think at all, particularly with regard to use of resuscitation. Everybody gets resuscitated unless it is practically tattooed on your forehead or your attorney and your physician are at your bedside with legal documents in their hands at the time of your demise to prevent someone for instituting CPR. You could have every single organ system in total shutdown mode and they would still pump on your chest if you hadn't dated the paperwork properly. And resuscitation doesn't even work that well in the vast majority of people.[16]

CPR might get us breathing again, but then what—and *for* what?

In 1974, when my Uncle Dru was fifty-four years old, he had some chest pains. He was admitted to the hospital for tests and while on the treadmill he had a massive heart attack. It was Code Blue. With CPR they got his heart beating, but oxygen had been lost to the brain and he lived for seven years in a vegetative state. My aunt said that once in a while he would babble, and she thinks that one time she heard him say, "Die me."

The last time I saw him he was skin and bones and tied down to the bed. He had a feeding tube he did not like and he kept pulling it out, they said. When his kidneys started to fail, my aunt finally said, "Please remove the feeding tube." Until that moment my aunt didn't have the confidence to speak up, and during the entire process no one gave her a choice.

Sadly, hospice didn't receive its rightful respect or funding until 1982, which means my adorable Uncle Dru had his heart attack eight years too soon. Or, if he had had it before 1969, he would not have been "brought back to life" and would never have been tied down to a bed.

If your heart stops in a hospital, CPR will be done to you even if you are very frail and very sick and even if you have a directive that says DNR—because as Dr. Overton says, clinicians don't have time to find your paperwork. This procedure is done and that sets you on a course of all that modern medicine has to offer, which is a lot!

---

16 Margaret Overton, *Hope for a Cool Pillow* (San Francisco: Outpost 19, 2016), 35.

This teaches me that medicine is in charge of me when I am under its roof. Having learned this, I have decided that this is not what I want and I don't think it's what God wants for me. CPR is just one of the "miracle" procedures that are available to us today and I use it here as a metaphor for the entire bundle of offerings.

Stop trusting other people to save you.
Do not think too highly of them;
they are only humans who have not stopped breathing yet.
— Isaiah 2:22, ERV

The Goliath We Call Modern Medicine

According to the Kaiser Family Foundation analysis of 2017 OECD (Organization for Economic Co-operation and Development) data, as would be expected, wealthy countries like the US tend to spend more per person on healthcare and related expenses than lower income countries. However, even as a high-income country, the US spends more per person on health than comparable countries. Health spending per person in the US was $10,348 in 2016—31 percent higher than Switzerland, the next highest per capita spender.

While the significance of numbers these days tends to get lost in a time when the government talks in terms of trillions like it's pocket change, in the case of healthcare, what are we getting for our money? I wrote about the answer in my last book:

Some call this the Medical Industrial Complex. David Goldhill writes in his book *Catastrophic Care,* "In America there are approximately one million physicians in forty-one specialties, 5,754 hospitals, 12,751 FDA-approved prescription pharmaceuticals, and several hundred thousand Class III medical devices all treating 14,568 possible diagnoses in 310 million patients. . . . Medicare sets six billion individual prices."

Modern medicine for most of us starts with the physician who writes prescriptions and orders tests, who might send us to the hospital or to an assisted living place for rehab after an injury.

Think of nurses and other highly trained medical specialists. In 2014 there were 2.7 million Registered Nurses in the US. Modern medicine needs nurse practitioners, physical and occupational therapists, physician assistants, phlebotomists, clinical laboratory technicians, diagnostic medical stenographers, respiratory therapists, substance abuse counselors, epidemiologists, practical and licensed vocational nurses, medical assistants, medical equipment technicians, clinical social workers, medical secretaries, radiologic technologists, home health aides, personal care aides, surgical technologists, nursing aides, pharmacy technicians, paramedics, mental health counselors, and more. Think of all the buildings involved. This includes hospitals, doctor's offices, rehab facilities, out-patient clinics, nursing homes, and long-term psychiatric residential treatment centers.

Think of drugs and medical devices. They are developed and they go through rigorous approval processes then are marketed to physicians and to us directly. Some refer to this part of modern medicine as Big Pharma. It is a nickname for the Pharmaceutical Research and Manufacturers of America, which shortened is called PhRMA. Big Pharma works hard to innovate, lobby Congress, pay the fees associated with its regulating body, the US Food and Drug Administration (FDA), and to sell its ideas.[17]

What is modern medicine up to? Dr. Elisabeth Rosenthal, a physician turned journalist, says, "The American healthcare system is rigged against you."[18] If you are afraid of the cost of care and what it will do to your pocketbook, I suggest you read her book *An American Sickness: How Healthcare Became Big Business and How You Can Take It Back.* In the homework, I will take you through some exercises to help you provide direction about how you want your assets to be utilized as you become frail or seriously ill. Dr. Rosenthal's discoveries explain why Dr. Overton says that hospitals are immoral. Decisions are made by balance sheets, not by what is best for a patient.

The Doctors of Madison Avenue

Let's look at what is "sick," and who is "sick." Did you know that obesity was not considered a disease until 2013? What happens when a certain condition is designated as a disease? Money flows to treatments. My Grandmother Bryant was always round, but I don't recall anyone saying she was obese, I never heard her say she was on a diet, and I'm positive she was never treated by a doctor for obesity. Had she gone to the doctor, he probably would have scolded her for dipping snuff. As far as I could tell, this and her daily RC Cola were her big vices. She lived to be eighty-two, and that seems like a fine age to die.

We are sicker and more medicalized than ever, due to the fact there are more definitions of "sick," and that the definitions of "sick" change to benefit the people we have to pay to take care of us.

What defines "sick"? Modern medicine defines "sick," and it is very good at telling us what "sick" looks like, with specific measurements it takes for us—and it

---

17 Hattie Bryant, *I'll Have It My Way* (Houston: Bright Sky Press, 2015), 147–148.
18 Rosenthal, *An American Sickness*, 241.

conveniently changes the definition and even makes up diseases. Would my father have ever been told he had low-T? My guess is that as he aged, he considered it normal to have less energy, less sex drive, and less muscle-building ability.

This table shows the effect of lower diagnostic thresholds on osteoporosis, high blood pressure, high cholesterol and diabetes.[19] The good intentions of professional societies to find and treat illness by lowering the threshold value for diagnosis opens the door wide to increased drug use.

HEALTHY REDEFINED OR WHO MOVED THE GOAL LINE?							
Osteoporosis in Women	*then*	8,010,000	*now*	14,791,000	=	6,781,000 more sick people
High Blood Pressure	*then*	38,690,000	*now*	52,180,000	=	13,490,000 more sick people
High Cholesterol	*then*	49,480,000	*now*	92,127,000	=	42,647,000 more sick people
Diabetes	*then*	11,697,000	*now*	13,378,000	=	1,681,000 more sick people

By changing the definition of healthy, millions more are medicalized.

What about our tendency to believe the medical marketing hoisted on us? Are there billboards around your town telling you to come to this or that hospital? Do you receive direct mail from the hospitals and physician groups who want your business? Do you ever wonder why these messages are presented to us? What about Big Pharma and its power to persuade? In 2016 pharmaceutical companies spent $5.6 billion on direct-to-consumer advertising,[20] to convince us that we need what they have. In that same year, we spent $450 billion on what they told us to buy,[21] for diseases they told us we might have. Projections are that we will spend $610 billion in 2021.[22] Is our pill-popping lazy? Could this possibly track with a spiritual laziness or a gradual decline over the centuries in our interest in spiritual formation?

On top of that, our affluence has increased our sugar consumption and it allows us to sit more than any human beings in history have ever been able to sit. In fact, it's

---

19 H. Gilbert Welch, Lisa M. Schwartz, and Steven Woloshin, *Over-Diagnosed: Making People Sick in the Pursuit of Health* (Boston: Beacon Press, 2011), 23.

20 Kevin McCaffey, "Drugmakers again boost DTC spending, to $5.6 in 2016," March 3, 2017, accessed September 10, 2017,https://www.mmm-online.com/home/channel/commercial/drugmakers-again-boost-dtc-spending-to-5-6-billion-in-2016

21 Pharmaceutical Commerce, "US drug 2016 sales, at $450 billion, moderate to single-digit growth," May 4, 2017, accessed September 10, 2017, http://pharmaceuticalcommerce.com/latest-news/us-drug-2016-sales-450-billion-moderate-single-digit-growth/

22 Bil Berkrot, "U.S. prescription drug spending as high as $610 billion by 2021," May 4, 2017, accessed September 10, 2017, https://www.reuters.com/article/us-usa-drugspending-quintilesims/u-s-prescription-drug-spending-as-high-as-610-billion-by-2021-report-idUSKBN1800BU

so bad for us that sitting is now called "the new smoking."[23] Then there's stress. Our own personal choices are at the root of most of our sickness, but we don't see it that way, and we can afford to depend upon others to fix us. Rather than schedule a walk, we schedule a doctor appointment.

Why does advertising work so well on us? We like the easy way, and we love the new shiny object. Choosing the easy way has made us soft, and our children are even softer than us. We are affluent, do everything we can to live bubble-wrapped lives, and invite our children to join us.

The ICU, under a Microscope

The ICU provides the front edge of medicine and is the most scientifically and technologically advanced department in a hospital. If our kidneys fail we can get our blood washed; if we can't swallow, a feeding tube is inserted; if we can't breathe, a "trach" is inserted to attach us to a breathing machine; and if our heart or lungs are failing, we can get Extracorporeal Membrane Oxygenation (ECMO). "This is to keep a patient alive until he recovers from an acute illness or can receive an organ transplant."[24]

Dr. Laura Morrison, professor and board-certified internist, geriatrician, and hospice and palliative physician at Yale-New Haven Hospital, told me, "The decades-long experiment we've been running to medicalize living and dying has failed us, as it often keeps us from having meaning all the way to the end. Our system is set up for us to all die in ICU. I think it is due to our inability to have the hard discussion and more skillfully and intentionally integrate technology and progress into the natural rhythm of our life cycle."

Is it possible that Dr. Morrison sees the ICU as our way of avoiding the inevitable? As Christians, we are using medical science to avoid what God has for us. Does our plastic faith melt under the lights of the ICU? In the ICU, we can pretend that our white-coat gods are in charge, while we shake our fist at heaven and put our foot down to stay in this flawed and broken world just because it's what we know. In the end, there is no escaping the fact that our time is limited. As the following chart shows, three of the major causes of death have their own timetable, and while they vary—and some beat the odds—eventually, we all end up at the zero axis.

---

23 Ryan Fiorenzi, "Sitting is the New Smoking," September 25, 2018, accessed November 27, 2018, https://www.startstanding.org/sitting-new-smoking/
24 Jessica Nutick Zitter, *Extreme Measures* (New York: Avery, 2017), 305.

HOW PEOPLE DIE[25]

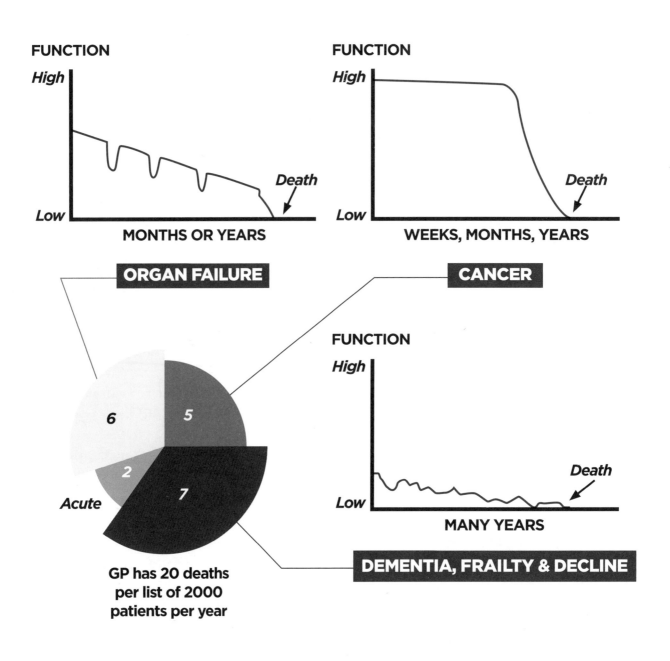

25 Scott A. Murray, "Interfacing palliative care with other disease specialties," lecture at Our Lady's Hospice Annual Conference—Moving Points in Palliative Care: Crossing Boundaries, Dublin, Ireland, March 4, 2010. Permission to use these charts was granted by Dr. Murray by personal communication September 18, 2014. In this chart GP refers to a general practitioner or a primary care physician.

Surrender to Prayer

ICU physician Dr. Jessica Zitter, in a lecture delivered to clinicians, said, "Technology in the hands of physicians often is the source of suffering and patients need to understand that surrendering is not the same as giving up."[26] Isn't surrendering exactly what we all did when we invited the Lord of the Universe to take over our lives? We are to surrender to the entire gospel, and that means let go and let God have his way every day, all the time, even and especially when it's time to surrender this physical body.

As Christians, when we surrendered to God, it included surrendering our misplaced faith in the religion of modern medicine. God's very first commandment to us was, "Thou shalt put no other gods before me." Our belief in medicine as religion will inevitably fail, but not before it makes us sick and blind to what Jesus came to give us: his very breath that never stops, as it breathes eternity into what will become our glorified bodies.

American Christians—and for sure, this is an American problem—have become so secularized when it comes to medicine that we don't even realize we are acting like those who have no faith. We might even take pride in our knowledge of medicine, and when a loved one becomes sick we gird ourselves with notebooks and file folders to brace for the battle ahead. Certainly, we have a responsibility to learn all we can about our illness, but when it fails to inform our thinking we tell the doctor to "just keep piling on of all of your technologies and drugs," or "doctor shop 'til we drop" to find one more angle, one more intervention, one more creative way to avoid the reality of our own mortality.

But what happens when the cardiologist, oncologist, pulmonologist, nephrologist, or intensivist (or any other hospital-based specialist who is dealing with life-limiting disease) says, "There is nothing more we can do"? We have just run into the terrifying reality that we've placed all our eggs in medicine's basket and just learned that the plan we had for a miracle is not going to hatch. Do we panic and become even more anxious and stressed, making ourselves even sicker with worry? Or, do we look elsewhere for guidance, where followers of God have gone since the beginning of time, to the one true and only Great Physician himself?

Moses and Hezekiah prayed and changed God's mind. While Moses was up on the mountaintop receiving the Ten Commandments written by God's finger in stone tablets, the four million Israelites under his leadership grew restless, and convinced Aaron that they needed a new god to worship; Aaron capitulated. God became so angry that he told Moses that the punishment for their disobedience was their total destruction. Moses thought quickly and talked God out of that idea (Exodus 32:7–14). We have to imagine that Moses had family and friends whom he loved, and that he fought for their lives right there on the spot.

---

26 Jessica Zitter, lecture, 2nd Annual Spirituality and Health Conference, October 11, 2017, San Antonio, TX.

In another example, Isaiah came to Hezekiah and told him that the Lord had sent him to tell him, "Set your house in order, for you shall die and not live." Hezekiah fell to weeping and pleading with God to let him live. He turned himself into the wall and wailed. He reminded God through bitter tears that he had walked faithfully and had done what was good in God's eyes, and for his obedience, God relented and allowed him to live (Isaiah 38:1–20, KJV).

The big prayers through the ages remind us that prayer is about listening to God as much as talking. We have to get all of this ourselves. We have to get it into our minds and hearts and the marrow of our bones. Think of it this way: It's just you and God. That's all. Medicine has an end. There is no end to God.

The problem with conflating modern medicine with the power of the Great Physician is that modern medicine becomes our crutch, our safety net just in case God doesn't hear us. Maybe we don't have the faith of Moses or Hezekiah, or we refuse to listen when God's answer is: No, you're not staying here. I'm taking you home.

In 1 Corinthians 3:9, Paul writes that we are co-laborers with God. We are to take part in our healing by doing what is good for our bodies and by praying that God guide the clinicians. At the same time, there will be an end to the medical interventions we are chasing when our lives are only full of modern medicine.

We often forget the most powerful weapon we have against disease and our own anxiety: the power of prayer. Pastor Tim Keller tells us when we're anxious, worried, or stressed, we need to work on the hard questions rather than run to what the world offers. He writes, "But Paul says, 'Whatever is true, whatever is noble, whatever is right, whatever is pure, whatever is lovely, whatever is admirable . . . think about such things. . . . And the God of peace will be with you' (Phil. 4:8–9). In effect he is saying: 'Think!' God made the world and we turned from him—but he's come back to save us at infinite cost to himself. And some day he will put everything right and we will live with him forever. If you really understood and believed that, nothing could get you down for long. So think. If you are discouraged, think about and take hold of Christian doctrine until it puts some health and peace into you."[27]

As Christians, we have the Word to lead the way as we think about the sensible use of modern medicine. Tim Keller is telling us to work on the deep spiritual questions and problems that may cause us to worry over ourselves. Christians are human, so we get depressed and discouraged. Our hearts get broken, our confidence runs out, and in a medical crisis it's easy to default to the fallible offerings of modern medicine when we know that the Great Physician provides greater and deeper healing. Let's use modern medicine in small doses and load up on what feeds our forever self, our souls. Marinate

27 Tim Keller, "Why Studying Doctrine Is the Best Medicine," *The Gospel Coalition,* March 18, 2013, accessed June 20, 2018, https://www.thegospelcoalition.org/article/why-studying-doctrine-is-the-best-medicine.

in God's Word. Meditate on it, memorize it, wake up with it, go to sleep with it. Give your worries and problems over to the One who made you, who saved you and who is willing, if you let him, to bring you day-by-day closer to the perfection he has planned for you.

Data shows that older people do the majority of spending when it comes to medicine. It's as if we hit that magic number when Medicare kicks in and all of a sudden, whatever treatment we might want is free! Certainly to a large degree, we earned it, and it is reasonable to avail oneself of the wonders of modern medicine. All too often, we forget the deeper healing that he has promised and put our faith exclusively in modern medicine. Medicine is science. We can trust it as real. As for God? Well, we think we believe.

Franciscan friar, priest, and author Richard Rohr, says, "Many people never grow up or remain narcissistic into their old age."[28] He writes that we live in an adolescent culture caught up in success and security while denying the opportunity for our own personal growth and wisdom to blossom. Stuck there, we'll always be afraid, uncomfortable with ambiguity and worse, we'll keep depending on what we can see and hear and taste and touch when God tells us to put all of our trust in him and him alone.

Wise thinkers and leaders like Charles Spurgeon, the "Prince of Preachers" said, "It is impossible that any ill should happen to the man who is beloved of the Lord; the most crushing calamities can only shorten his journey and hasten him to his reward. Ill to him is not ill, but only good in a mysterious form. Losses enrich him, sickness is his medicine, reproach is his honor, death is his gain. No evil in the strict sense of the word can happen to him, for everything is overruled for good. Happy is he who is in such a case. He is secure where others are in peril, he lives where others die." Spurgeon also reminds us, "The fear of God is the death of every other fear; like a mighty lion. It chases all other fears away."[29] Billy Graham writes, "We may be old in years, but if our faith is immature, we will enter those latter years fearful and unprepared."[30] He also famously wrote, "You're born. You suffer. You die. Fortunately, there's a loophole."[31]

Here's something else the great Charles Spurgeon had to say about illness and death: If we really believe in miracles, then we must give God the chance to deliver, while always remembering and trusting in the fact that sometimes God's choice is to bring the sick into their perfect healing that only happens with him. In 2002 Billy Graham told of how two years earlier he was in the hospital and thought he was dying. He prayed, "Lord, I'm a sinner, I need you. I need your peace." Dr. Graham said God answered and gave him a peace unlike he had ever known, and he did not pass over to heaven until 2018.[32]

---

28 Richard Rohr, *Falling Upward* (San Francisco: Jossey-Bass, 2011), 3.
29 Charles Spurgeon, *The Treasury of David,* Vol. 2 (Peabody, MA: Hendrickson, 1988), 93.
30 Billy Graham, *Nearing Home* (Nashville: Thomas Nelson, 2011), 151.
31 Matthew Boffey, "In Loving Honor: 12 Quotes on Evangelism from Billy Graham," February 21, 2018, accessed July 4, 2018, https://blog.logos.com/2018/02/ loving-honor-12-quotes-evangelism-billy-graham/
32 Billy Graham Memorial Newsroom, accessed July 4, 2018, https://demoss.com/newsrooms/ billygraham/background/quotes-by-billy-graham.

The Power of Prayer

Let's enter every situation with prayer. Let's do this now before we are sick or frail. We are to pray. Don't assume the worst is cast in stone. Don't assume you'll die soon when medicine struggles with curing you. Pray. But, don't expect medicine to be the healer when it has tried what it knows and has failed. Making this shift will change completely the trajectory of your care and how you spend the last years, weeks, and days of your life.

Invite your prayer partners to come to your home and pray and let God heal. God doesn't need modern medicine. God made you, God can heal you. You will learn from my essay in the appendix "My Directive in Essay Form" that while I'm not into the technologies of medicine, I'll take the pain medication every time and hope to be at home when I take it.

"What you want, when you want, how you want" is the prayer I learned from Tim Keller. Then I add, "Father, you know what I want, and I actually believe that you gave me this particular desire so here goes: I want to be healed. I want my fully functioning life back!" Rick Warren taught me that yelling at God is OK because God can take it. My translation of Lamentations 2:19 is this: "Get up and pray for help. Pray every hour on the hour. Lift up your hands and pour out your feelings like water in prayer to the Lord." Yes, God is OK with me screaming at the stars. You should try it. It wears you out, then you fall into God's arms to sleep.

My dad prayed for twenty years that my mom would be healed of her mental illness and Dad got a "no," but hardly anyone knew about my dad's praying. Kay and Rick Warren prayed for twenty-seven years that God would heal their son of his mental illness. God didn't give them a "yes" to that prayer, and their son committed suicide in April of 2013. This is the most public "no" to faithful prayer I know about. The whole world watched as Kay and Rick suffered. I have sent dozens of friends to his sermon series, "Getting Through What You're Going Through." I have spent hours and hours with these sermons myself. It's how I learned to lament.

As Christians we must memorize that there is no end to God's power. There's power to heal and power to take us out of here.

Richard Foster's book *Celebration of Discipline: The Path to Spiritual Growth* has sold more than 1 million copies. He writes, "We are working with God to determine the future! Certain things will happen in history if we pray rightly. We are to change the world by prayer."[33]

---

33 Richard Foster, *Celebration of Discipline: The Path to Spiritual Growth* (New York: Harper Collins, 1978), 35.

Prayers and Belief Work

My dear friend Betsy speaks about her own healing experience, and I asked her to write it so that I could share it with you. It is a testament to faith, perseverance, hope, and the power of prayer:

As a bit of background for my story of how I was healed from Stage IV cancer, I should say that I grew up in a Christian home and have had very good health most of my life. From an early age, I memorized many verses from the Bible through the years. By the time I was 14 years old I had had two genuine experiences when I heard God speaking to me in my spirit, not audibly to my natural ear.

During 1995, I was working full-time in community relations for a large corporation, enjoying working with the numerous grant requests, assisting the manager of the corporate philanthropic program. I began to notice back pain that year in August, began taking Tylenol on a regular basis, thinking the issue would clear up in a few weeks, but it did not.

So, I scheduled an appointment with my doctor (OB/GYN) in October. The ultrasound was completed, and I received a call from my doctor whom I knew very well on a Friday afternoon. His words were both a shock and a blessing. He said, "I believe you have a serious issue which will require an immediate biopsy which I have scheduled for Tuesday morning. However, I know you are a Christian as I am, and I want you to remember this: doctors practice medicine, but only God heals." I replied, "Thank you, and yes, I do believe the same thing!"

The biopsy revealed I had non-Hodgkins cancer. Further tests revealed I was in Stage IV, very serious indeed. I was referred to an oncologist, but at my first visit, I sensed in my spirit two important facts: he was quite arrogant in the way he presented his plan of treatment and did not appreciate my questions. So, I asked two nurses I knew personally to tell me about other oncologists they knew.

The second doctor I met was a perfect fit for me. She was compassionate, was not offended that I wanted to be a "partner" in choosing the action protocol. Also, she appreciated the fact that I was a person who relied on God and prayer; she confirmed that she also was a believer. The plan was to be very aggressive, and in layman's terms, chemo treatments would be given 5 days in a row, every 21 days.

After going home and praying, I frankly told the Lord in prayer that I wanted Him to guide me through every step. First, He impressed a scripture on my heart, Romans 8:11: "If the same Spirit which raised Jesus from death dwells in you, He shall quicken your mortal body." Next, He impressed on me that I must read Psalm 103 three times a day as though it were part of my prescriptions. I am a "speed reader" generally when I read silently, but when I began reading, immediately I heard God say, "No, I mean read it aloud." Aha! I already knew there is a verse that says, "Faith comes by hearing the Word of God."

Next, as I arrived for my first chemo treatment, the nurse and I visited a bit, and I shared my plan to pray over everything, including her and the medicine. She also confirmed she was a believer in God's word. From Matthew 16:18, I prayed that even if I consumed any deadly thing, it should not harm me. The papers I signed to give permission for treatment were very sobering to me; basic terms said doctors would calculate chemo in quantities that would kill half of the cancer cells without killing me! There would be nine periods of treatment. Okay, I got started at the end of October, 15 days after diagnosis. Praying aloud three times a day and giving thanks for every pill, every IV, etc.

After 5 months, my oncologist was not satisfied with my progress, so she referred me to MD Anderson in Houston. Thankfully, they accepted me with the idea that I was a candidate for bone marrow transplant. They adjusted the protocol as well, stronger chemo. A very interesting result from the test on my bone marrow: they found NO cancer cells. The tumors in my lymph glands were still there, but the bone marrow was clear. They decided to test me again in 3 months, and if it was still clear, they would take a harvest from me (eliminating the risk of rejection). In June 1996, they harvested my bone marrow and put it in the bank for future use.

I continued the new chemo protocol and the praying aloud three times a day till I went back to MD Anderson in March 1997. That day, the doctor said, "I wish I could tell everyone what I'm telling you today. All the tests we've just done confirm that you have experienced a spontaneous remission. You have no evidence of cancer cells anywhere in your body."

Wow! I asked if that happened very often, and she said I was the first one she had that year, March 21. Further, she said there was no scar tissue where the biopsies were taken, very unusual. Both I and my husband thanked her for overseeing my treatment. She said I would need to have re-checks every 90 days for 2 years, so I did that, continuing to pray aloud daily. Every test revealed that I was still free of cancer. Next, I was checked every year for 5 years, and still free of cancer.

When I get the opportunity to share my story, I emphasize that no matter what the doctors say, please inquire of the Lord. Pray. Ask Him to guide you with His word. Give thanks over your medicines, and get an agreement with the doctors that you can ask questions along the way if you have any. Try to find a doctor that believes in the power of prayer.

In March of 2017, yes, I am still free of cancer. I have not ever needed the bone marrow transplant. Praise to God Almighty!

Betsy Bilbruck
Mandeville, Louisiana

Richard Foster and Dallas Willard were lifelong friends. Both would be considered giants of our faith, thought leaders, writers, and formidable leaders in spiritual formation. Mr. Foster and Dr. Willard were prayer partners for decades, and in 2013 God took Dr. Willard home at the age of seventy-seven. There is no way for me to know what prayers were offered for Dr. Willard's healing, but I do know this: Dr. Willard's body of work helped millions of Christians deepen their faith, and the theologians and scholars who spoke at his funeral should have been able to pray Dr. Willard well if we go by their curriculum vitae. brief auto-biographical sketch

Only seventy-seven years old? We mutter to ourselves, "That is way too young to die, I'm going to live to be a hundred!" What did Dallas Willard say about death? He didn't believe in it. "Jesus made a special point of saying those who rely on him and have received the kind of life that flows in him and in God will never experience death. . . . Jesus shows his apprentices how to live in the light of the fact that they will *never* stop living."[34]

There was a woman who spent twelve years going to doctors and she spent every penny she had searching for a cure. She suffered a great deal under the care of many physicians and just got worse. She heard about a new kind of physician who was going to be close enough to home that just maybe she could get into see him. Even though

---

34 Gary W. Moon, ed., *Eternal Living: Reflections on Dallas Willard's Teaching on Faith and Formation* (Downers Grove, IL: InterVarsity, 2015), 239.

Hattie Bryant

there was a big crowd trying to see this man, she pressed through and got close. At the moment her hand touched his clothing, her bleeding stopped. It was Jesus himself who said simply to her, "Your faith has healed you" (Matthew 9:20–22; Mark 5:25–34; Luke 8:43–48, NIV). Oh, I so want to hear Jesus say this to me.

> *Death is no more than passing from one room into another. But there's a difference for me, you know. Because in that other room I shall be able to see.*[35]
>
> — Helen Keller

---

[35] Joseph M. Demakis, *The Ultimate Book of Quotations* (Raleigh, NC: Lulu Enterprises, Inc., 2012), 70

Learn the Limits
of Modern Medicine

Big Word for This Session: SEEK

The mind governed by the flesh is death, but the mind governed
by the Spirit is life and peace.
— ROMANS 8:6-7, NIV

Far better to take refuge in God than to trust people.
— PSALM 118:8, MSG

Opening

Optional Listening: "It Is Well," accessed through illhaveitgodsway.com/biblestudy

Opening Prayer: Father God, show us fresh insight now, as we open ourselves to you. We ask this humbly in the name of Jesus, Amen.

Take some time to discuss the homework. Was there anything in the questions or readings that was especially interesting or impactful?

 ## Play the Session Two video.
Available on the DVD or from the link found on this page:
illhaveitgodsway.com/biblestudy

Video Discussion

The money spent on healthcare tells us that we believe in it with our whole wallet. Recent reporting shows that Medicare spent $170 billion on patients' last six months of life.[36] This does not take into account the hard dollars spent by families, and some go bankrupt before the loved one dies. Our full-court press to keep another person alive, and often ignore their own wishes, is mostly a result of our lack of confidence in God's great plan and maybe even selfishness. The $170 billion did not save a life; it prolonged the dying process.

1. What are some ads you have seen that make big promises?

2. How should we think about those ads and all that modern medicine has to offer? Read aloud Romans 12:2 (MSG):

   "Don't be so well-adjusted to your culture that you fit into it
   without even thinking. Instead, fix your attention on God. You'll
   be changed from the inside out. Readily recognize what he wants
   from you, and quickly respond to it. Unlike the culture around you,
   always dragging you down to its level of immaturity God brings the
   best out of you, develops well-formed maturity in you."

 Play the FAQ video "Why Wouldn't I Want Everything Medicine Has to Offer?"
Available on the DVD or from the link found on this page:
illhaveitgodsway/biblestudy

---

36 Kaiser Health News, "End-of-Life Care: A Challenge In Terms of Cost And Quality," June 4, 2013, accessed October 10, 2017, https://khn.org/morning-breakout/end-of-life-care-17/

Going Deeper

Christopher Bogosh is a nurse and a pastor who has spent years taking care of dying patients. He writes in *Compassionate Jesus* that Christians worship at the altar of medicine because. . . .

- We are afraid to die.
- We are addicted to this world and love our lives in it.
- We are absorbed in worldly attitudes about modern medicine without questioning its value, truth, ethics, or goals.
- We see modern medicine as neutral.
- We have a low or confused view of God's providence.[37]

Mr. Bogosh also says, "The 'theology' of medicine does not believe in your soul."[38]

Here's why he says this: Today there are three dominant worldviews.

- Naturalism/Realism. The visible is all there is.
- Nirvana. The world is an illusion. The real world is we are all one.
- Theism. God is all-knowing and all-loving.

3. In which worldview do you think modern medicine "hangs out"? How does this worldview limit modern medicine?

4. Read Matthew 6:33 and Psalm 23 out loud, then complete the blanks below:

Matthew 6:33 *what we worry about ← eat, drink, what I wear*

Seek God and get what?
I get _all these things_.

What do these verses mean to you?

When I kept my mind focused on God's truth I am being transformed and I am able to be at peace find rest and have hope

Psalm 23

Claim God and get what?
I get _all I desire_.

rest, refreshment, restoration of my soul, leading paths of righteousness, His presence w/ me in the valley and through it, His protection + provision, His anointing Goodness + mercy are with me all the days of my life

37 Christopher Bogosh, *Compassionate Jesus* (Grand Rapids, MI: Reformation Heritage Books, 2013), 26-27.
38 Christopher Bogosh, telephone interview with the author, October 19, 2017.

5. Now, read Joshua 1:8 and Psalm 1:1-4 out loud, and again complete the blanks below:

Joshua 1:8
Meditate on God and get what?
I get _prosperity + good succe_

Psalm 1:1-4
Meditate on God and get what?
I get _lasting good fruit_ .
all that I do prospers

How would you restate the message of these two verses, in your own words?

Here's my translation: The one who meditates on God will not wither. Or: The one who depends on God will never fade, die, be removed, lose a leaf, nor do anything but prosper.

Seek God, meditate on God, listen to God, commit to God, and you live now in The Kingdom of God. Your spirit is already in heaven now. There is no distance between you and your creator and Savior. *None.* "Seek" means "look." Open your eyes to the invisible life here. You'll gain a childlike aura that can take years of stress off of your face and out of your body (more about that in session 5)! No waiting to get rid of the physical body. You get all of God now if you really want him.

6. Read Matthew 6:10 aloud. How do we get God's will?
We ask God   Read His word, His instruction
                     Meditate   "   given in Scripture
                     Rom 12:2

7. What *is* God's Kingdom?

8. What does Dallas Willard say we are (see page 25)?
... never ceasing spiritual beings with an unique eternal destiny to count for good in God's great universe

9. How does this definition of humankind help us understand the Word of God?

Please read Matthew 4:4. Jesus had been fasting for forty days, and the devil himself shows up and tells Jesus to turn the stones into bread. Famously, "Jesus told him, 'No! For the Scriptures tell us that bread won't feed men's souls: obedience to every word of God is what we need'" (TLB). Or you may know the translation "Man shall not live by bread alone" (KJV).

10. What do you think this means? If we are theists, not naturalists, or if we are Christian and not agnostic, what is Jesus saying?

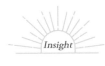
Insight

To me, this means we can't depend upon the physical to make our life work. Yes, we need food and water. Yes, we like chocolate, too. Jesus seems to be boldly warning us not to depend upon what we think makes us healthy.

11. Bread, as in flour, will only provide limited aid. What is bread a metaphor for?

Here are just a few suggestions; you'll likely come up with others:

Bread = Money. We can't buy happiness or a cure, if a cure doesn't exist.
Bread = Modern Medicine. Medicine will only provide limited solutions.
Bread = A beautiful house. Things break.
Bread = The right clothes. They go out of style.
Bread = A busy schedule. A temporary sense of self-importance.

Do you think we can agree that Jesus is saying man cannot live by anything physical alone? This includes "man shall not live by medicine alone." Man shall not depend upon, or expect modern medicine alone, to save him from the heartache of this life and the diseases we've piled upon ourselves since creation.

12. Jesus says, "The kingdom of heaven is at hand" (Matthew 4:17, KJV). What do you think this means?

13. What does this mean to you, and how could this change your view of sickness?

Let's go back to Newton and the change that happened when science took over defining our lives. When there were so few explanations of how things work, we depended upon God to direct, inspire, and provide. Now we simply don't need God until we get to the end of our rope—or in the case of this study, the end of modern medicine.

We have to seek God, because God wants us to want him. He wants us, loves us, sees our potential but he will not force himself on us. If he took away our free will, he would be taking away what makes us in his image. His Spirit, put in us by God himself, has to rise up and take over. We have to ask it to move us, lead us, coach us, comfort us, teach us. This is the Spirit Isaac Newton killed off, kicking the door open for the scientists to rule the world, thereby paving the way for the gods of medicine to grab hold of our hearts.

14. Do we find the Kingdom of God in modern medicine? How does this affect the way you think about what is being offered to you by medicine?

Hattie Bryant

15. Dr. Kreeft said, "The medieval mind was primitive in its science but profound in its theology. The modern mind is the reverse." Do you think your theology is primitive?

16. How is it that we are so good at living lives that skim the surface? What would a mature theology get us?

17. Here's a theologically mature statement: Physical health should not be our primary goal. How do we know that this is true?

18. What advice does Tim Keller give us for dealing with our addiction to this life and all that modern medicine has to offer? (See page 42.)

19. Let's stop and have a look at ways we can interact with modern medicine when
    we become frail or seriously ill. The American Bar Association Commission on Law
    and Aging toolkit helps us think about how we want our end-of-days preparation
    to go. (This exercise is used with permission.) Curative care is what we think of
    as medicine—treatments, medication, monitoring, surgery, etc. Comfort care is
    palliative medicine, which we'll discuss more in detail in the next session.
    It is important to know that many treatments can keep us alive, even when there
    is no chance that the treatment will reverse or improve our condition.

Ask yourselves what you would want in each situation described if the treatment
would not reverse or improve your condition. We give you these five ways to
describe your wishes so please circle the number that best fits you. The group can do
this together and discuss answers.

WHAT IF YOU...	WANT CURATIVE CARE			WANT COMFORT CARE	
No longer can recognize or interact with family or friends.	1	2	3	4	5
Comment _____					
No longer can talk clearly.	1	2	3	4	5
Comment _____					
No longer can respond to commands or requests.	1	2	3	4	5
Comment _____					
No longer can walk but can get around in a wheelchair.	1	2	3	4	5
Comment _____					
Are in severe pain most of the time.	1	2	3	4	5
Comment _____					

Hattie Bryant

Are in severe discomfort (such as
nausea, diarrhea) most of the time.   **1   2   3   4   5**

Comment _____

Are on a feeding tube to keep you alive. **1   2   3   4   5**

Comment _____

Are on kidney dialysis machine
to keep you alive.   **1   2   3   4   5**

Comment _____

Are on a breathing machine
to keep you alive.   **1   2   3   4   5**

Comment _____

Need someone to care for you
24 hours a day.   **1   2   3   4   5**

Comment _____

No longer can control your bladder.   **1   2   3   4   5**

Comment _____

No longer can control your bowels.   **1   2   3   4   5**

Comment _____

Live in a nursing home permanently.   **1   2   3   4   5**

Comment _____

Other   **1   2   3   4   5**

Explain _____

Now, read the following questions and check the box that best reflects your response.

	STOP CURATIVE TREATMENT AND PROVIDE COMFORT CARE/PALLIATIVE CARE TO ALLOW NATURAL DEATH	PROCEED WITH AGGRESSIVE TREATMENTS
What would you tell your doctor to do if you had a disease that was incurable and you would become dependent on others for your care?		
What would you tell your doctor to do if you had a disease with no hope of improvement and you were suffering with severe pain?		

Father, help us see what you want us to see. Dispel any fears or anxieties we have about our own death and the death of those we love. Set us free! In Christ's name we ask, Amen.

Before the next group session, complete the following homework and Reading 3.

HOMEWORK

The Cost of Care

1. How can optimism be our enemy when it comes to engaging with modern medicine?

2. Please look up the words of Jesus found in Matthew 6:21 and write them here.

3. Please write here how you have thought about modern medicine in the past, and now how you might be learning to see it in a new light. Be ready to share your answers with the group during your next session.

You now know that money drives all of modern medicine. Patients and families often pay a high price—psychologically and economically—for difficult and unscripted deaths. Since writing *I'll Have It My Way,* so many have come up to me to tell their sad stories of loss, not just about losing a loved one but about entire families being financially destroyed by a protracted illness. In most all of these stories there's a recurring theme that goes like this: "If my father knew what we were spending to keep him 'alive,' he would rise up out of his bed and tell us to leave him alone and let him die in peace."

Too many of the frail and seriously ill who are not strong enough to speak for themselves are being "kept alive" by a well-meaning family. Dr. Richard Della Penna, who was responsible for the care of millions when he was the chief medical officer for senior care for a huge healthcare system, sounds the alarm:

> Care at the end of life is expensive and all too often has no effect on function, independence, duration or quality of life. Furthermore it can cause more pain and suffering with no chance of improving anything. The fact that costs are insulated makes the technology and ineffective care even more alluring.

The Truth of the Cost
Think through the following questions and be prepared to share your answers with the group during the next session.

4. Do you think that if you spend a lot of money on a person you love, this means that they are receiving the best care?

5. Does spending money on a loved one keep you from feeling guilty?

6. Do you spend to avoid someone thinking that you didn't do everything possible?

7. Since you and all of your loved ones paid your insurance premiums for years and paid into the Medicare system, do you feel entitled to everything modern medicine has to offer—even if it won't help you? Or do you think, "It's worth a try. I paid for it"? Or, do you just accept all that a physician offers?

8. Share any stories (without names!) of families you have seen struggle with the cost of caring for loved one.

9. Modern medicine has much to offer, and yet it is extraordinarily expensive and time-consuming. This is your chance now to create a financial planning tool and prevent a burden being left on your loved ones, which could arise when you become seriously ill or frail.

Check the statement that fits you best:

☐ It's OK with me if keeping me alive requires unlimited resources paid for by insurance (private/Medicaid/Medicare), my own savings/the savings of family, and makes heavy demands on the time and emotions of family and friends.

☐ It's OK with me if keeping me alive requires unlimited resources paid for by insurance (private/Medicaid/Medicare) and my own savings. However, I do not want my care to be a financial or emotional burden on my family. So, when my money runs out, let me go naturally. I realize that this choice means I might have nothing left to leave to my children and grandchildren.

☐ It's OK to keep me alive so long as it's paid for by insurance (private/Medicaid/Medicare). So, when my benefits run out, let me go naturally. That way I can leave any assets to my family.

☐ I am beginning to understand that keeping me alive at all costs (money and the efforts required of so many others) is not what I want for my life. I want to leave gently with people sorry to see me go rather than hoping I will go.

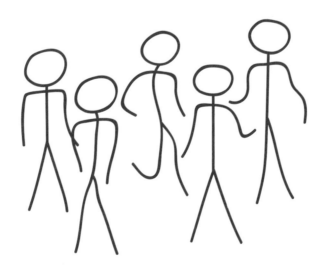

My dad was good at facing the truth about money, because he never had much of it. He grew up poor and wouldn't tolerate waste in our house. He was a conservationist, and today we might call him an environmentalist. At seventy-eight he had cancer, and the chemotherapy was a drag. He could see that it was a short-term fix, and he considered the time and money being spent on him to be a bad investment. He announced to us, "Save the healthcare for the grandchildren." He invited hospice in and slipped away peacefully, taking time to have some nice conversations.

10. Why do you think most of us say, "I don't want to be a burden" but then don't have the courage to be honest with our families about money? *"There is no 'ransom' that can buy you out of death [Psa 49:7-12]. It is coming, and it will strip you of everything dear to you. It is then, utterly foolish to live your life as if economic prosperity could keep you truly safe or as if you will never die. Only God can give you things of value that death cannot Touch that but only enhance." Tim Keller, Songs of Jesus, p 103*

11. Why is knowing the Word of God good for our health? Can prayer be God's medicine? Can worship be God's medicine? Can community with other Christians be God's medicine?

12. Can God's medicine kill pain? Kill depression? Kill cancer? Explain your answers.

13. How did Helen Keller describe what death will be like (see page 48)?

Verse for meditation:

Matthew 6:33 (NLT): Seek the Kingdom of God above all else, and live righteously, and he will give you everything you need.

While the world runs unquestioning into the arms of modern medicine, we can run into the arms of our Savior who showed us how to live and how to die.

Verse for meditation:

1 Corinthians 2:12 (CEV): God has given us his Spirit. That's why we don't think the same way that the people of the world think.

Before the next session, be sure to complete Reading 3 on pages 65–75. You can also review the Session Two videos at illhaveitgodsway.com/biblestudy.

There's a Gentle Path

Accept That We Are Not God and We Will All Die
Learn the Limits of Modern Medicine
Understand Our Healthcare Choices
Choose a Proxy and Provide Specific Instructions
Start Living in God's Kingdom Now

Jesus said, "I am leaving you with a gift—peace of mind and heart.
And the peace I give is a gift the world cannot give.
So don't be troubled or afraid."
— JOHN 14:27, NLT

John Eldredge, author, counselor, and lecturer on Christianity, writes in his best-selling book, *Wild at Heart*, "The most dangerous man on earth is the man who has reckoned with his own death. All men die; few men ever really live. Sure, you can create a safe life for yourself . . . and end your days in a rest home babbling on about some forgotten misfortune. I'd rather go down swinging. Besides, the less we are trying to 'save ourselves,' the more effective a warrior we will be."[39]

Few of us can picture ourselves as warriors, especially when faced with a serious illness or the end of life. It's far easier to wave the white flag, resigned to be captives of modern medicine's conquest over our bodies and healthcare choices. The brave will fight back, and it will take courage that can only come from God. The choices can look reckless to those around us who prefer to live a safe life and want you to play it safe, too. Be on guard; the ones closest to you can play on your heart strings, and have the ability to take your focus off heaven.

> Take the case of courage. No quality has ever so much addled the brains and tangled the definitions of merely rational sages. Courage is almost a contradiction in terms. It means a strong desire to live taking the form of a readiness to die. . . . He must seek his life in a spirit of furious indifference to it; he must desire life like water and yet drink death like wine.[40]

Our Leaving Is a Worship Experience

During a Sunday sermon, my pastor stated, "We have to do everything afraid." He was preaching about doing the hard things, and referred us to Daniel and the dangerous life he led in Babylon. He referred us to Nehemiah, the man who led Jewish exiles out of Babylon to rebuild the walls of Jerusalem. While God may not give us such hard assignments as Daniel and Nehemiah, we will all face death. It's going to be difficult if we don't get ready, and far easier if we do.

How do we choose just exactly the way we want to live all the way to heaven? How do we make our last days our best days? How do we demonstrate God's glory all through a life-limiting illness or extreme frailty? How do we make our death a worship experience?

Mr. Eldredge wrote this about his dear friend. "As Craig was making the hard decision to leave treatment down in Houston, and return home for what he knew would be the end, he said, 'I don't want to die fighting cancer; I want to die loving

---

39 John Eldredge, *Wild at Heart: Discovering the Secret of a Man's Soul* (Nashville: Thomas Nelson, 2011), 171.
40 G. K. Chesterton, *Orthodoxy*, (London: William Clowes and Sons, 1908), accessed June 15, 2018, https://www.gutenberg.org/files/16769/16769-h/16769-h.htm.

people.' On the first of August, at 6:30 a.m. Craig took his last breath, and exhaled. It had been a still morning; at that moment a wind blew into the house, lifting the curtains, swirling around the room for more than thirty minutes. Holy. So holy."[41]

My friend named Mark told me something similar about his mom's death. He said he heard the air move, and there was no window open; and then he saw a tiny flash of light. Mark is a banker and not an elegant writer like Mr. Eldredge but Mark's face as he told about his mom's death told me that he'd had a worship experience. Hospice nurses have told me that they know when the angels come.

Dr. John Morley, one of America's most important geriatricians and just one of the many physicians who helped me write *I'll Have It My Way*, tells a moving story about one of his patients. The woman was ninety-four years old and in what he considered to be good health. She called him to come to her side as she told him that she would die shortly. She lived in a nursing home where Dr. Morley was the attending physician, and he was surprised that she had decided her death was imminent. He recalls that he sat down, took her hand, and that the two spoke for about thirty minutes talking casually about their lives. He writes, "Her hand slipped out of mine and she was silent. There was a feeling of warmth in the room and then I thought I saw a blinding light fly out of the window. I felt more at peace than I ever had."[42]

H. Fischer-Hullstrung was the physician attending as the Nazis executed Dietrich Bonhoeffer (1906–1945) by hanging. This man had no idea who Bonhoeffer was, but later wrote about his last five minutes, "In the almost fifty years that I worked as a doctor, I have hardly ever seen a man die so entirely submissive to the will of God."[43]

A missionary to India, Amy Wilson Carmichael, writes of the worship experience she had while watching a child go to God:

> Her name was Lulla. She was five years old, a Brahman child of much promise. She had sickened suddenly with an illness which we knew from the first must be dangerous. We could not ask a medical missionary to leave his hospital, a day and a half distant, for the sake of one child, but we did the best we could. We sent an urgent message to a medical evangelist trained at Neyyoor, who lived nearer, and he came at once. He arrived an hour too late.
>
> But before he came we had seen this. It was in that chilly hour between night and morning. A lantern burned firmly in the room where Lulla lay; there was nothing in that darkened room to account for what we saw. The

---

41 John Eldredge, "We Live Forever," August 22, 2016, accessed November 2, 2017, https://www.ransomedheart.com/blogs/john/we-live-forever
42 John Morley, "Is There a Good Death?" LinkedIn, January 12, 2018, accessed March 20, 2018, https://www.linkedin.com/pulse/good-death-dr-john-morley/.
43 Eric Mataxas, *Bonhoeffer: Pastor, Martyr, Prophet, Spy* (Nashville: Thomas Nelson, 2010), 532.

child was in pain, struggling for breath, turning to us for what we could not give. I left her with Mabel Wade and Ponnamal, and, going to a side room, cried to our Father to take her quickly.

I was not more than a minute away, but when I returned she was radiant. Her little lovely face was lighted with amazement and happiness. She was looking up and clapping her hands as delighted children do. When she saw me she stretched out her arms and flung them around my neck, as though saying good-bye, in a hurry to be gone; then she turned to the others in the same eager way, and then again, holding out her arms to someone whom we could not see, she clapped her hands.

Had only one of us seen this, I think, we might have doubted. But we all three saw it. There was no trace of pain in her face. She was never to taste pain again. We saw nothing in that dear child's face but unimaginable delight.

We looked where she was looking, almost thinking that we would see what she saw. What must the fountain of joy be if the spray from the edge of the pool can be like that? When we turned the next bend of the road, and the sorrow that waited there met us, we were comforted, words cannot tell how tenderly, by this that we had seen when we followed the child almost to the border of the Land of Joy. [44]

How can we die in an utter state of submission to the one true God who awaits us? How can we make our death a worship experience for all who are present—not just the last five minutes but the last few years, months, weeks, and days? One woman learned from her mother's death that "Dying doesn't cause suffering. Resistance to dying does."[45] We can't see God or others he is sending to get us if we're fighting to stay here. And, we deny others the opportunity to experience the peace that he offers to all. Far better that, as we leave those around us, they step back and watch grace happen. Let all see what our great God does for those who trust him.

What the Doctors Know That We Don't

We are clay jars holding a treasure. We are the receivers of the living water that flows from the infinite to us and through us, the receivers of sacred breath that never stops and keeps us in perfect peace and prays for us. We have the sacred breath of creation only humans receive: then the breath Jesus promises to us, the one he called comforter;

---

44 Amy Wilson Carmichael, *Gold Cord* (Fort Washington, PA: CLC Publications), 18.
45 Terry Tempest Williams, *Refuges: An Unnatural History of Family and Place* (New York: Vintage Books, 1992), 53.

Hattie Bryant

the force that counsels, prays, teaches, inspires: the birth breath and the re-birth breath are ours as believers. Paul admonishes us when he writes, "Don't you realize that your bodies are actually parts of Christ . . . that your body is the temple of the Holy Spirit, who lives in you and was given to you by God?" (1 Corinthians 6:15, 18, NLT).

Doctors know better than any that we are all little clay jars. After all, for doctors, "death is just another day at the office."[46] They also know the system in which they work and it changes the way they think and act when it comes to their personal illnesses.

Joe Gallo, MD, MPH, is the director of The Johns Hopkins Precursors Study. He asked 765 older physicians about end-of-life care. He discovered first that 64 percent of them had advance care plans in writing, compared to only 26 percent of the general population. He also asked them: "If you had brain damage or some brain disease that cannot be reversed and makes you unable to recognize people or speak understandably, but you have no terminal illness, and you live in this condition for a long time, indicate your wishes regarding the use of each of the following medical procedures."[47]

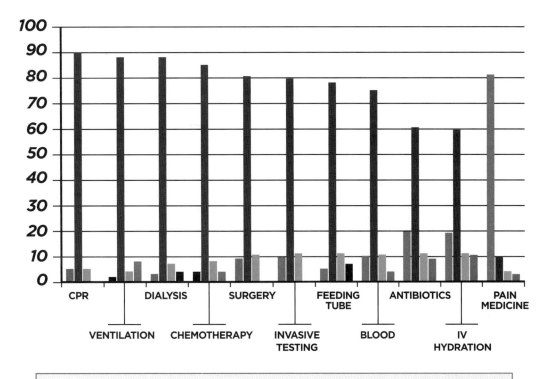

YES, I WOULD WANT ### NO, I WOULD NOT WANT
UNDECIDED ### TRIAL, BUT STOP IF NO CLEAR IMPROVEMENT

46 Haider Warraich, *Modern Death* (New York: St. Martin's Press, 2017), 212.
47 J. J. Gallo, et al., "Stability of Preferences for End-of-Life Treatment After 3 Years of Follow-Up," *JAMA Internal Medicine* 168 No. 19 (2008): 2125–2130.

I'll Have It God's Way

Why would physicians turn down these modern medicine options, especially when these are the same ones they would recommend if it were *us*? They understand that the results of these treatments will not get them the kind of lives they want to live. My own research for my book told me what physicians thought of these end-of-life treatments:

- CPR: "futile, odds aren't good"
- Ventilation: "no hole cut in throat, but could intubate for a few days"
- Dialysis: "chronic malaise, fatigue, nausea, blood pressure going up and down"
- Chemotherapy: "vomiting, weakness and it doesn't always work; question everything"
- Surgery: "I'd rather not; need to know the purpose, the stats"
- Invasive Testing: "from surgery to drawing blood; depends"
- Feeding Tube: "not for me"
- Blood: "maybe one transfusion, but no more; do not want to depend upon it having to be repeated"
- Antibiotics: "if I am comatose or have lost my mind and I get an infection, just kiss me goodbye"
- IV Hydration: "no thanks, unless it's just to get me over a non-serious illness"

Many families of the seriously ill tell doctors, "Keep my mom alive. We're going to pray for a miracle." This is after the doctors have explained that they have done everything they know to do and nothing is working. My mom's doctor told me that there was nothing more that could be done for her. She didn't know us, couldn't move, couldn't communicate, couldn't swallow, and required a manmade hormone to keep her kidneys functioning. We were confident that mom would not want to be kept alive with a feeding tube and medication only to lie in a bed in a comatose state for weeks, months, or even years. We had been praying for five weeks, and it was clear to us that our God wanted her with him.

The Real Physician

Jesus spent about one-third of his ministry in healthcare. You can read in the New Testament about the thirty-one individual healings and the twenty references to mass healings. There was the leper in Galilee, the servant of the Roman Centurion, Peter's mother-in-law sick with fever, the paralytic at Capernaum, a deaf man, an epileptic, Jairus' daughter, the man at the pool of Bethesda, and the man born blind. We only get to read about the few of many Jesus healed during his ministry.

Jesus knew his power to heal and also knew that even his days on earth were numbered. Rather than leave his followers then and us today without hope, he said, "I tell you the truth, anyone who believes in me will do the same works I have done, and even greater works, because I am going to be with the Father" (John 14:12, NLT). Modern medicine does in fact achieve "greater works," thanks to the medicines and technology that Jesus didn't have at his disposal. In the case of making the blind to see, Jesus used mud, spit, and prayer and healed a few. Today, The Mercy Ships operate a fleet of hospital ships bringing modern medicine to developing countries. Thousands of people who were once blind due to cataracts have their sight restored by ophthalmologists who perform a twenty-minute surgical procedure, fulfilling one of the immortal lines from "Amazing Grace": "was blind, but now I see."

It is true that doctors today perform what appear to be miracles by modern standards. Organs are replaced, tumors are shrunk, blood pressures are lowered, and broken minds pieced back together so the afflicted can function within our society. We are not wrong to want to be healed. God created the doctors, nurses, pharmacists, technologists, and all the medical professionals who perform these miracles every day. The problem is that we lay persons simply do not understand the serious implications of telling modern medicine to "do everything to keep my mom alive," when the chances of her recovery due the nature of her illness are very slim. Let's say mom has suffered a severe stroke and exhibits no brain activity. For the medical staff, "everything" can mean permanent intubation or a tracheostomy (to breathe for her) and a percutaneous endoscopic gastrostomy (PEG) inserted (to feed her).

In addition to numerous complications with both procedures, this is a signal to the hospital that the patient needs to be released, usually because Medicare and Medicaid won't cover these conditions in a hospital setting. So, like it or not, mom gets moved to a nursing home or other long-term care facility where she will spend the rest of her days confined to a bed—a situation that can go on for years. In short, "doing everything to keep my mom alive" often gives your mom a life of suffering. She may not be in physical pain, but the suffering will be spiritual, emotional, and psychological. So, if you are ever faced with the choice for someone you love, remember what Jesus said: "*I am the resurrection and the life. The one who believes in me will live, even though they die; and whoever lives by believing in me will never die*" (John 11:25–26, NIV, emphasis added). This was the authority and power granted only to him by the Father, not the medical professionals ready to do everything to save us.

What Gives Life Meaning?

Rather than as a way to be kept alive no matter what, we need to think of medicine as beneficial until what is offered keeps our life from having meaning. That is very personal. Gregg Allman, the singer-songwriter and member of the Allman Brothers, had tumors in his liver. Doctors told him they could not cure the liver cancer, but they could shrink the tumors with radiation that could damage his vocal chords. He had already decided that his life would be without meaning if he could not sing and play his guitar all the way to the end, so he said no. His days on earth were reduced, but life for him continued to have meaning because he was able to sing until he died.

Remember Craig who made the hard decision to leave treatment at MD Anderson Cancer Center and return home for what he knew would be the end? His friend says that he was a man who loved God and loved people, so when he said, "I don't want to die fighting cancer; I want to die loving people," it was no surprise to those who knew him. His friends who were with him for the last time were able to say, "Craig, you *won*. In everything that is important, you *won*."[48]

Another man whose sister was in the ICU knew that she did not like being stuck in bed, and even less with the breathing tube the doctors had inserted. She couldn't speak but was able to communicate that she wanted out of the situation she was in. Knowing his sister's wishes, the brother asked the doctors to remove the breathing tube. He trusted that God would provide the final answer; either she would breathe on her own, or God would take her home to be with him. One day after the breathing tube was removed, that is exactly what God did. Had the brother not made this decision and entrusted his sister into God's hands, doctors would have cut a hole in his sister's throat to be permanently attached to breathing machine.

Being Smart Medical Consumers

When a doctor gives you a difficult diagnosis there is a very good chance they are not telling you all of the truth about the seriousness and the difficulty you will face. Research tells us that doctors put a positive spin on what they tell us, and sadly, money figures into the "truth-telling" equation. Hospitals are companies in the healing business—some more compassionate than others, but ultimately, all depend on money to survive. One physician writes, "As long as someone stands to profit from the propagation of health services, which may or may not improve your life most particularly at the end of your life, you cannot trust that you will receive sound advice."[49] This helps explain why people are deluded into thinking that the suffering they endure in the hope of a cure is all about them. The truth is that all that money— and the more the better—spent on futile treatment mostly benefits the bottom line of modern medicine. Not only do we have no idea what these services really cost, but, from our lack of due diligence, we continue to tolerate high prices and poor service from healthcare that we wouldn't tolerate from any other market segment. We must learn to treat healthcare as the big "C" consumer with choices and power—and not act like gullible sheep being sold a bill of goods.

Difficult diagnoses are tests in sheep's clothing. Without a test there's no testimony. Without tests we don't know our strength. Rick Warren says that God

---

48 Eldredge, "We Live Forever."
49 Overton, *Hope for a Cool Pillow*, 157.

is not so interested in what we do as he is in who we are. Sitting in worship at Saddleback Church, I have no idea how many times I have heard Rick Warren say, "This is not heaven. This is a broken world. Everything is broken. Our bodies are broken, our relationships are broken, our hearts are broken. Only Jesus can fix us." God builds our character and our faith through an ongoing series of tests and problems, and somehow he ensures that these are lifetime companions.

We have a choice: Insist that doctors busy themselves with activity that is medically futile and rob us of what matters most to us; or, be about the work that God has planned for us to do all along. This is our last time to be salt and light. This is our last time to bear witness to the power we have in us that was placed in us by God himself. We have the promise of eternal life, so why spend time getting treatments and procedures when doctors tell us they won't work, or discover that doctors do what they do for money or to make themselves feel important? Instead, when you hear a difficult diagnosis, we need to be brave and ask our physician:

1. Please describe this diagnosis in detail, so I can understand what this means to me.
2. What is the typical trajectory of this disease?
3. What happens if I do not take treatment for this but opt for palliative medicine now?
4. What are the treatment choices?
5. Can I speak with others who have already dealt with these options?

When the diagnosis comes, let's go back to Paul when he writes in Philippians 4:8–9 (MSG), "I'd say you'll do best by filling your minds and meditating on things true, noble, reputable, authentic, compelling, gracious—the best, not the worst; the beautiful, not the ugly; things to praise, not things to curse. Put into practice what you learned from me, what you heard and saw and realized. Do that, and God, who makes everything work together, will work you into his most excellent harmonies." That last phrase in the NIV says "And the God of peace will be with you."

Depend more than ever now on your "go-to" scriptures when you are hit with news you do not want to hear. Here are a few of my favorites. Try putting them in first person and make them a conversation between you and God, otherwise known as prayer:

> *Exodus 14:14* The LORD will fight for me and I will be at peace.
> *Deuteronomy 31:8* The LORD goes before me; he is with me; he will not fail me, he will not drop me or leave me, I am not to fear or be dismayed no matter what I see happening with my eyes.
> *Psalm 23* The LORD is my shepherd….
> *Psalm 25:8-10* You promise if I trust you LORD, you will personally instruct me.
> *Psalm 34:4* I sought the LORD and he delivered me from all my fears.

Psalm 46:10 I am to be still, and know that God is God and I am not.

Psalm 55:22 I cast my burden on the LORD.

Psalm 61:2-3 Lead me to the rock that is higher than I.

Psalm 73:23-26 You hold me by the right hand, you guide me with your counsel, you are bringing me to glory. Whom have I in heaven but you? And there is nothing on earth that I desire besides you. My flesh and my heart may fail, but you, Father God, are the strength of my heart and my portion forever.

Psalm 91:14-16 If I hold your hand, Father, you will get me out of trouble and you will give me the best of care. Since I know and trust you, no matter what time it is, when I call you answer.

Isaiah 41:10 I am not afraid or dismayed because my God is here. He is giving me strength right now, and he is helping me right now.

Jeremiah 29:11 I know you have plans for me to prosper, Father.

Matthew 28:11 You will give me rest and peace in my soul.

2 Corinthians 4:6 God you have put your light in my heart. . . .

1 John 3:1 I am your child.

1 John 4:4 You are greater than any of my problems.

Revelation 21:4 He will wipe away every tear from my eyes, and death shall be no more, neither shall there be mourning, nor crying, nor pain anymore, for the old way of doing things is gone.

Songs work wonders on the spirit. Sing them loud, especially when you are alone in the car or in the morning shower.

- On Christ the solid rock I stand; all other ground is sinking sand.
- Lord I run to you; no one else will do.
- In Christ alone I place my trust, and find my glory in the power of the cross.
- Jesus gave her water, and it was not from the well.
- Great is thy faithfulness, oh God my Father.

Call on all of your heaven songs now:

- On Jordan's stormy banks I stand and cast a wishful eye.
- On heaven's shore I fix my compass . . . oh the glory there like a jewel so rare, joy forever more there on heaven's shore.
- Ain't no grave can hold my body down.
- Swing down chariot come and let me ride; rock me Lord, nice and easy. I've got a home on the other side.
- Take my hand, precious Lord. Lead me home.
- This world is not my home; I'm just a passin' through.

74   Hattie Bryant

Before I get frail or hear a difficult diagnosis, I want to be ready to say, "not as I will." I want to be that strong and graceful oak tree planted for God's glory (Isaiah 61:3). I want to be the tree planted by still waters with deep roots in God, a tree that doesn't feel heat or drought (Jeremiah 17:8).

Our little broken jar of clay has fallen apart. It has lost its shape and wants to decay and go back to dirt. If we let go and let God, we can trust him to keep his promise. As the clay crumbles away, the treasure it has been holding from the moment we invited Jesus in is released to God himself. He is waiting to make us perfect and he will.

All of my life I have been trying to stay in the boat with Jesus, and I imagine him calling me to get out and walk on the water to him when he's ready for me to shake free from this body. I'm the thief on the cross, and Jesus promised, "today you will be with me in paradise" (Luke 23:43, NIV).

SESSION THREE

Understand Our Healthcare Choices

Big Word for This Session: COURAGE

Don't be afraid, for I am with you. Don't be discouraged,
for I am your God. I will strengthen you and help you.
I will hold you up with my victorious right hand.
— ISAIAH 41:10, (NLT)

Opening

Optional Listening: "Precious Lord," link found at illhaveitgodsway.com/biblestudy

Opening Prayer: Father God, show us fresh insight now, as we open ourselves to you. We ask this humbly in the name of Jesus, Amen.

Take some time to discuss the homework and readings. Share and discuss your answers from the questions under "The Truth of the Cost" on page 60.

Play the Session Three video.

Available on the DVD or from the link found on this page: illhaveitgodsway.com/biblestudy

Video Discussion

1. How did 911 change the dying process?

2. What did Dr. Murray's physician friend do when he heard his own difficult diagnosis?

3. Do doctors tell us the unvarnished truth? How can we decide what to do if we don't have the truth about our condition?

4. Why do you think we are not allowed to say, "I'm dying," but we're cheered on when we say, "I'm fighting this disease?"

Most Americans don't want to sort out healthcare choices so they simply do what doctors tell them to do. This is the reason as many as 80 percent are dying in institutions. Fear is underlying the sequence of events that brings so many to the kind of death they never wanted for themselves. Thinking about our soul is a waste of time for modern medicine so as we defer to modern medicine we break the first two commandments.

Hattie Bryant

Instead, our thoughts should reflect those of Paul in Romans 8:5-6 (NIV): "Those who live according to the flesh have their minds set on what the flesh desires; but those who live in accordance with the Spirit have their minds set on what the Spirit desires. The mind governed by the flesh is death, but the mind governed by the Spirit is life and peace."

Going Deeper

May we be like the great evangelist, Dwight Moody (1837–1899), who said:

> Some day you will read in the papers that D.L. Moody, of East Northfield is dead. Don't you believe a word of it! At that moment I shall be more alive than I am now. I shall have gone up higher, that is all—out of this old clay tenement into a house that is immortal; a body that death cannot touch, that sin cannot taint, a body fashioned like unto his glorious body. I was born of the flesh in 1837. I was born of the spirit in 1856. That which is born of the flesh may die. That which is born of the spirit will live forever.[50]

5. Discuss the story of Dietrich Bonhoeffer on page 67.

Bonhoeffer had it easy, right? You might say in that he was never sick and died a martyr at the age of thirty-nine. He never got frail or seriously ill, and never had to make decisions about what treatment to take or not take. But in a sermon Bonhoeffer preached in London before he was thrown into a Nazi prison, we learn that he was prepared for what we would call a cruel ending:

> Whether we are young or old makes no difference. What are twenty or thirty or fifty years in the sight of God? And which of us knows how near he or she may already be to the goal? That life only really begins when it ends here on earth, that all that is here is only the prologue before the curtain goes up—that is for young and old alike to think about. Why are we so afraid when we think about death? . . . Death is only dreadful for those who live in dread and fear of it. Death is not wild and terrible, if only we can be still and hold fast to God's Word. Death is not bitter, if we have not become bitter ourselves. Death is grace, the greatest gift that God gives to people who believe in him. Death is mild, death is sweet and

---

50 Quoted in Steve Mays, *Overcoming* (Ventura, CA: Regal, 2012), 55.

gentle; it beckons to us with heavenly power, if only we realize that it is the gateway to our homeland, the tabernacle of joy, the everlasting kingdom of peace.[51]

6. What would it take for you to get where Bonhoeffer was when he wrote this? How can you make your death a worship experience for all who are present? Not just the last five minutes but the last few years, months, weeks, and days?

Have my mind set on things above and being transformed by the renewing of my mind

Communication with physicians can be difficult because they say things that we often misinterpret. This poor communication is at the root of the cause of much needless suffering at the hands of modern medicine.

Words Don't Mean the Same Thing

When you arrive for the next discussion with your doctor, do not assume that you will understand one word the doctor says. While they speak English, they speak it as it is used and taught in medical school.

They say: **Acute**

| You think: Serious, will kill me. | They think: This just popped up; it is not chronic. |

They say: **Treatment**

| You think: Cure. | They think: process/procedure/protocol/usual intervention. |

They say: **Adverse drug reaction**

| You think: I'll get a rash. | They think: you could end up dead/in the hospital/this has a wide range of meanings, can run the gamut; no intent to indicate severity only thinking of the cause. |

They say: **Perhaps**

| You think: Of course. | They think: maybe but more likely not. |

---

51 Otto Dudzus, *Bonheoffer for a New Generation* (London: SCM Press, 1986), 140.

Hattie Bryant

They say: **We can try**

You think: It will work.

They think: It is technically possible to do this but there is no suggestion of success.

They say: **We can enroll you in a study**

You think: Great. I'm going to get cutting-edge treatment!

They think: You fit the criteria we are seeking for the research. You want to participate in order to add to medical knowledge.

They say: **We know a little**

You think: They know more than they are telling me.

They think: This is totally experimental with no proven long-term positive results.

They say: **Adjuvant therapy**

You think: I have no idea.

They think: What we'll do after we have done surgery chemotherapy and/or radiation.

They say: **Your cancer has responded to the chemotherapy**

You think: I am going to be cured.

They think: There has been some effect on the tumor.

7. Does anyone have personal experience with friends or family who were too optimistic about physician reports? Does this help to explain why lay people may be confused as they enter into treatment for a serious illness?

If you ever have to go the hospital, YOU have to be prepared to manage your care.

Modern medicine looks like the picture on the next page. When you have a serious illness or suffer a trauma that lands you in the hospital, as many as a dozen physicians could be involved in your case. They each will know some aspect of your case, as they have test results that guide them to assess and address the problem they are trained to fix. They are time-pressured by today's medical environment, so they won't have much time to talk with you, or even with the other physicians who are on your case. You are lost in the complexity, and so is your family.

How do we get on the gentle path if physicians are not interested in talking about it as an option?

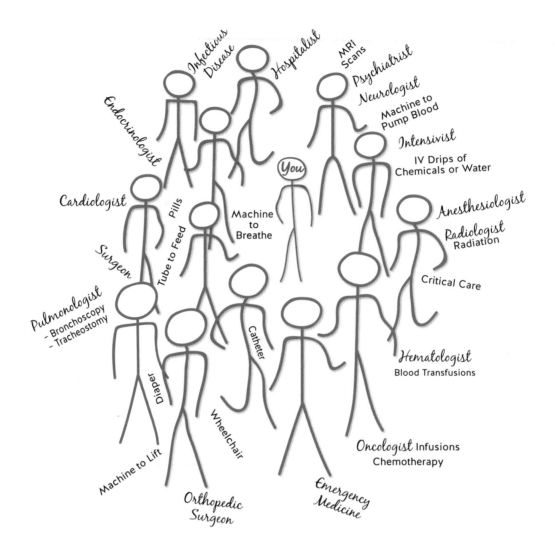

The figure shows many stick figures surrounding a central one labeled "You," each labeled with a medical specialty or intervention: Infectious Disease, Hospitalist, MRI Scans, Psychiatrist, Neurologist, Machine to Pump Blood, Intensivist, IV Drips of Chemicals or Water, Anesthesiologist, Radiologist, Radiation, Endocrinologist, Cardiologist, Pills, Tube to Feed, Machine to Breathe, Surgeon, Critical Care, Pulmonologist – Bronchoscopy – Tracheostomy, Diaper, Catheter, Hematologist Blood Transfusions, Machine to Lift, Wheelchair, Orthopedic Surgeon, Emergency Medicine, Oncologist Infusions Chemotherapy.

- Question everything.
- Pray.
- Learn what kind of palliative medicine is available where you live and demand it. (Most hospitals have someone designated to direct palliative care but if you are an outpatient, what can you do?)
- Find a primary care physician to guide you. Find a pastor or group of praying Christian friends to be in your Circle of Care (more about this in the next session).
- Check into all social services available to the sick and aging in your community.

Memorize this:

Palliative medicine is for anyone who has a serious illness and at any stage of the illness. It is not about death and dying! It is about tending to the whole hurting you—mind, body, and spirit.

Hattie Bryant

Think of palliative medicine not as the newest type of medicine but the oldest.

How is palliative medicine different from other medical specialties? A team, including a physician, nurse, social worker, chaplain—and sometimes a psychologist, nutritionist, pharmacist, and/or music therapist—works with you to relieve your suffering.

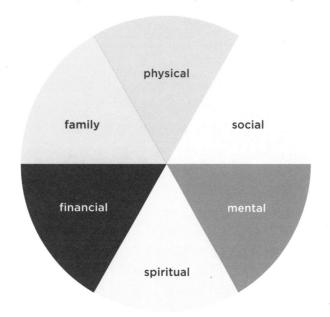

Palliative medicine looks at the whole you, not just the physical you. Read out loud these passages from Romans 8:

> The law always ended up being used as a Band-Aid on sin instead of a deep healing of it. And now what the law code asked for but we couldn't deliver is accomplished as we, instead of re-doubling our own efforts simply embrace what the Spirit is doing in us. (Romans 8:4, MSG)
>
> So now every righteous requirement of the law can be fulfilled through the Anointed One living his life in us. And we are free to live, not according to our flesh, but by the dynamic power of the Holy Spirit!
>
> Those who are motivated by the flesh only pursue what benefits themselves. But those who live by the impulses of the Holy Spirit are motivated to pursue spiritual realities. For the mind-set of the flesh is death, but the mind-set controlled by the Spirit finds life and peace.
>
> In fact, the mind-set focused on the flesh fights God's plan and refuses to submit to his direction, because it cannot! For no matter how hard they try, God finds no pleasure with those who are controlled by the flesh. (Romans 8:4–8, TPT)

8. What are we to do as Christians when we or loved ones are presented with a difficult diagnosis?

9. What is your greatest fear? Not being like everyone else? Poverty? Being alone? Seen as lazy or not willing to fight? Failure? Losing your mind? Dying before you finish your to-do or want-to list? A cancer diagnosis?

10. What are we to do with our fears?

Here we wade in deep, to prepare for the time when we do receive a difficult diagnosis, or when we become so frail that we need help with the activities of daily living.

Joseph Gallo, MD, professor at John Hopkins Bloomberg School of Public Health, and a group of his colleagues collected responses from 765 older physicians to learn how they felt about using life-sustaining treatments for themselves under the following scenario:

> "If you had brain damage or some brain disease that cannot be reversed and makes you unable to recognize people or to speak understandably, but you have no terminal illness, and you live in this condition for a long time, indicate your wishes regarding the use of each of the following medical procedures by placing a check mark in the appropriate column."[52]

11. Now, it's your turn. Please check the boxes on the following page that fit your response. If you like, you can review the physicians' answers on page 69.

---

52 J. J. Gallo, et al., "Stability of Preferences for End-of-Life Treatment After 3 Years of Follow-Up," *JAMA Internal Medicine* 168 No. 19 (2008): 2125–2130.

Hattie Bryant

PROCEDURE	YES, I WOULD WANT	NO, I WOULD NOT WANT	UNDECIDED	I WOULD WANT A TRIAL TREATMENT, BUT STOP IF NO CLEAR IMPROVEMENT
Cardiopulmonary resuscitation (CPR)		✓		
Mechanical ventilation		✓		
Intravenous hydration		✓		
Feeding tube (via mouth, trachea or into stomach) to provide nutrition		✓		
Major surgery		✓		
Dialysis		✓		
Chemotherapy for cancer		✓		
Invasive diagnostic testing such as endoscopy (equipment inserted in the body to examine an area)		✓		
Blood or blood products		✓		
Antibiotics		✓		
Pain medications, even if they dull consciousness and indirectly shorten my life				✓

12. If your health ever deteriorates due to a serious illness—and your doctors
    believe you will not be able to interact meaningfully with your family, friends or
    surroundings—check which of the following statements best describes what you'd
    like to tell them:

    ___✓___ I prefer that they stop all aggressive, life-sustaining treatments and
    allow natural death to come gently.

    _____ I would like them to keep trying life-sustaining efforts.

13. To take the lead when you hear a difficult diagnosis will take courage. Would you be afraid to question a physician? If yes, why?

14. What did we learn from Betsy? Please go back to pages 45–47 to review.
    a. Who did Betsy fire and why?
    b. What did she tell her new doctor?
    c. Did her new doctor believe in prayer?
    d. What did Betsy do over every pill and every treatment?
    e. When Betsy prayed for help, what did God give her?
    f. What did Betsy do three times a day for years?

To close your session, read through Psalm 103 as a group:

> Praise the LORD, my soul; all my inmost being, praise his holy name.
> Praise the LORD, my soul, and forget not all his benefits—who forgives all your sins and heals all your diseases, who redeems your life from the pit and crowns you with love and compassion, who satisfies your desires with good things so that your youth is renewed like the eagle's.
> The LORD works righteousness and justice for all the oppressed.
> He made it known his ways to Moses, his deeds to the people of Israel: The LORD is compassionate and gracious, slow to anger, abounding in love. He will not always accuse, nor will he harbor his anger forever; he does not treat us as our sins deserve or repay us according to our iniquities. For as high as the heavens are above the earth, so great is his love for those who fear him; as far as the east is from the west, so far has he removed our transgressions from us.
> As a father has compassion on his children, so the LORD has compassion on those who fear him; for he knows how we are formed, he remembers that we are dust. That life of mortals is like grass, they flourish like a flower of the field; the wind blows over it and it is gone, and its place remembers it no more. But from everlasting to everlasting the LORD's love is with those who fear him, and his righteousness with their children's children—with those who keep his covenant and remember to obey his precepts.
> The LORD has established his throne in heaven, and his kingdom rules over all.

Hattie Bryant

Praise the LORD, you his angels, you mighty ones who do his bidding who obey his word. Praise the LORD, all his heavenly hosts, you his servants who do his will. Praise the LORD, all his works everywhere in his dominion. Praise the LORD, my soul. (NIV)

Closing Prayer:

Father, help us see what you want us to see. Dispel any fears or anxieties we have about our own death and the death of those we love. Set us free! In Christ's name we ask, Amen.

Before the next group session, complete the following homework and Reading 4.

HOMEWORK

To get on and stay on the gentle path, you start by defining what a meaningful life is to you personally.

 ## Play the video "FAQ: What about out-of-pocket cost of care?"

Available on the DVD or from the link found on this page:
illhaveitgodsway.com/biblestudy

Physician and financial planner Dr. Carolyn McClanahan has a company called Life Planning Partners. The company tagline is "Financial Health for Life." She requires her clients to complete her checklist called "Quality of Life Requirements." I have included a version of this checklist below.

1. As you fill out this checklist, consider: What gives your life meaning and joy? For Gregg Allman, it was singing and playing his guitar. Add specifics on the blanks provided below. Gregg would have written, "To be able to sing."

In order to live the life you desire, it is important for you to retain the ability to: (Initial all that apply to you)

☐ Share your thoughts through words, gestures, or assistive devices.

☐ Understand what people are saying to you.

☐ Know that you are hungry. You are able to eat and swallow if someone feeds you.

☐ Chew and swallow food. Losing this ability results in the need of a feeding tube.

☐ Take care of your own toileting needs.

☐ Take a bath or shower with or without assistance.

☐ Interact in social settings.

Hattie Bryant

List other functions that are important to you:

_____

_____

_____

_____

_____

_____

In the appendix (pages 151–152), you will find another version of this, so you can make copies for your proxies and Circle of Care. This version includes instructions that if your healthcare providers state you will not regain the above functions, you are to be provided care that will keep you comfortable and pain-free until you die. If you'd like, once you have finished filling in all the blanks, you can also write your wishes in essay form. Flip to "My Directive in Essay Form" in the appendix on pages 140–142 for an example. I consider this a love letter to my family, friends, and physicians.

2. What are your biggest concerns and fears about being frail or seriously ill?

   alone

   Confinement

3. What are you looking forward to?

4. What goals are important to you now? How would those goals change if you were seriously ill?

"I say this with absolute confidence. If you practice what I'm telling you, keeps my word *you'll never have to look death in the face." (John 8:51, MSG)* see death

ADL activities of Daily living

5. How would deep belief in these words of Jesus change the last few years, months, weeks, and days of your life? *They will give me hope + encouragement*

6. How can we make our last days our best days? How can we make our death our last offer of praise to our Creator? *Dependence on God's Word. Prayer. Fellowship w/ the Saints*

7. Read 2 Corinthians 4:16. How can we create a worship experience for all who are by our side as we die? *Renewal of our inner man day by day*

8. What does it look like to die fighting cancer?

9. What does it look like to die loving people? *no guilt, no shame, forgiveness in my heart, love reigning*

10. We are clay jars holding a treasure. What is that treasure? *Truth of the Gospel*

We are the receivers of living water that flows from the infinite. We are the receivers of sacred breath that never stops and keeps us in perfect peace and prays for us. Read the following aloud:

> Don't you realize that your bodies are actually parts of Christ . . . that your body is the temple of the Holy Spirit, who lives in you and was given to you by God? You do not belong to yourself, for God bought you with a high price. So you must honor God with your body. (1 Corinthians 6:15, 19–20, NLT)

11. What does this mean to you now? What can it mean to you when you become frail or seriously ill?

12. When a doctor says, "there's nothing more we can do," are Christians hanging on these words of Jesus? "I tell you the truth, anyone who believes in me will do the same works I have done, and even greater works, because I am going to be with the Father" (John 14:12, NLT).

Do you imagine that God is in all aggressive care? Do you imagine that God expects us to accept all the treatments available? Do you really *have* to eat? (The answer to this last question is: No. Of course, eat if you are hungry for food; just remember that loss of appetite is natural.)

"I am the resurrection and the life. The one who believes in me will live, even though they die; and whoever lives by believing in me will never die" (John 11:25–26, NIV). There it is in black and white, a direct quote—and if your Bible has red letters, you read this in red and white.

13. Why is it so hard to die in America today?

Did you know that modern medicine is so confused about the definition of death that it has redefined life? A body permanently intubated, with no brain-wave activity, is considered by modern medicine to be alive.[53]

14. How will you balance your God-given desire to live and survive an illness (by accepting what medicine offers) with the need to accept that death could come sooner than expected? Or, how does this affect how you view the serious illness of loved ones?

53 Warraich, *Modern Death*, 134.

15. What about that hymn we have all sung hundreds of times?

> When we've been there ten thousand years,
> Bright shining as the sun,
> We've no less days to sing God's praise
> Than when we'd first begun.

What is it talking about? What is it speaking to you?

Eternal everlasting life. Going to be with Jesus in the place my heart has always longed for where I'll be with all I love and praise God forever.

16. If ten thousand years is just the beginning of our perfect life with God in our new and glorified body and free from our jar of clay, why do we fret over holding on for another year or two, or month or two, or week or two?

17. Please look up Psalm 90:10. Copy that here. *The years of our life are 70, or even by reason of strength 80; yet their span is but toil + trouble; they are soon gone, and we fly away.*

18. Are you letting others define you? Do you go along to get along? Explain.

What does it say in 1 Thessalonians 2:4b? "Our purpose is to please God, not people" (NLT). Or Exodus 23:2a (NIV): "Do not follow the crowd in doing wrong." We need to think and pray for ourselves, to protect ourselves from our culture.

19. Does it scare you right now to say out loud, "I am dying"? Why or why not?

It shouldn't scare us, as we are born "terminal," right? We're all dying right now.

20. Where does our courage come from? *from the spoken + read Word of God - Holy Spirit prayers + exhortation of other \ inspired believers*

Hattie Bryant

21. Think back to a time when you needed courage. What did you have to do, and how did you do it? *Set my mind on the Word of God Was a part of the Sunday night prayer group*

> *"What God has planned for people who love him is more than eyes have seen or ears have heard. It has never even entered our minds!" (1 Corinthians 2:9, CEV)*

22. What does this passage mean, in the context of this study? *The best is yet to come and I shall live happily ever after*

God tells us to do this: "Surrender your heart to God, turn to him in prayer, and give up your sins—even those you do in secret" (Job 11:13–14, CEV).

If we follow this command, we get this: "Then you won't be ashamed; you will be confident and fearless. Your troubles will go away like water beneath a bridge, and your darkest night will be brighter than noon. You will rest safe and secure, filled with hope and emptied of worry" (Job 11:15–18, CEV).

Verses to meditate on this week:

> *John 14:27 (NLT): I am leaving you with a gift—peace of mind and heart. And the peace I give is a gift the world cannot give. So don't be troubled or afraid.*

> *2 Timothy 1:7 (CEV): God's Spirit doesn't make cowards out of us. The Spirit gives us power, love, and self-control.*

Before the next session, be sure to complete Reading 4 on pages 95–103. You can also review the Session Three videos at illhaveitgodsway.com/biblestudy.

Create a Circle of Care

Accept That We Are Not God and We Will All Die
Learn the Limits of Modern Medicine
Understand Our Healthcare Choices
Choose a Proxy and Provide Specific Instructions
Start Living in God's Kingdom Now

Do not let your hearts be troubled. You believe in God; believe also in me. . . .
I go to prepare a place for you.
— JOHN 14:1–3, NIV

The Bible is a textbook for life, and one of its most difficult lessons is taught with clarity and conviction by the greatest teacher who ever lived:

Then Jesus began to tell them that the Son of Man must suffer many terrible things and be rejected by the elders, the leading priests, and the teachers of religious law. He would be killed, but three days later he would rise from the dead. As he talked about this openly with his disciples, Peter took him aside and began to reprimand him for saying such things.

Jesus turned around and looked at his disciples, then reprimanded Peter. "Get away from me, Satan!" he said. "You are seeing things merely from a human point of view, not from God's" (Mark 8:31–38, NLT).

Just one chapter later, Jesus tells his disciples again, "The Son of Man is going to be betrayed into the hands of his enemies. He will be killed but three days later he will rise from the dead" (Mark 9:31, NLT). Again, the disciples let it go in one ear and out the other.

For the third time, this time over a meal, Jesus tells his disciples that he is going die. Jesus is a poet, a painter of pictures, a storyteller, so he doesn't say, "I'm going to die soon." He said, "This is my body broken for you; do this in remembrance of me. . . . This is the new covenant in my blood, which is poured out for you. . . . [I] will go as it has been decreed" (Luke 22:19–20, 22, NIV).

Just after Jesus has said to the disciples that his body is broken and his blood is poured out, he goes to the Mount of Olives to pray. He only takes Peter, James, and John with him and invites them to pray, "so that you won't fall into temptation" (Luke 22:40, NIV). You probably remember that they didn't pray because they fell asleep, and we soon learn that Peter fell into temptation. When the powers that be came to arrest Jesus, Peter tried to stop the arrest by cutting off the ear of the servant of the high priest who was leading the mob.

Again, Jesus had to speak firmly to Peter, "Put your sword away! Shall I not drink the cup the Father has given me?" (John 18:11, NIV) It is fascinating that this is the same man who Jesus called "the rock [upon which] I will build my church, and the gates of hell will not prevail against it" (Matthew 16:18, ESV). Peter was using all of his might to keep Jesus from dying. Jesus wasn't intimidated by Peter; rather he put Peter in his place—and that's what we have to do.

Satan at the Bedside

This is a lesson with a warning: When God reveals to you that you are dying and you start telling the ones who love you the most, like Peter, they will not hear from you what they do not want to hear. Their grief and selfishness blind them from seeing your reality—and without them realizing it, your death becomes more about what is best for them and not you.

When we say to our family and friends, "I'm tired of struggling with disease. I want palliative care so that I can relax and enjoy as much time as I have left with you," they can pretend they didn't hear, tell us that they don't want to talk about it, or may succeed at shutting us down. When an emergency does arise, despite our wishes, they may insist on calling 911, which will trigger the continuation of more and more modern medicine and give you a "life" you never imagined or wanted that could go on for days, weeks, months, or even years.

Think about the Peters in your life. By thinking hard now and acting on what you're learning to do here, you will have a much better chance of living and dying the way you want—while lovingly but firmly showing the Peters in your life that you believe what Jesus has promised.

When it is our time to leave here, we can say nearly the same words that Jesus said. We can say to friends, family, and physicians. "I am going to be turned over to disease or frailty that will kill me then I will rise, too, and go to the place Jesus has prepared for me." The miracle is that we don't even have to wait in some dark spot for three days. We never leave the presence of God and will never see darkness again for all of eternity.

The Futility of a Long Death

"The cup" Jesus had to drink was death. Absent an accident that takes us immediately, we will have some sort of winding-down process before we die. Modern medicine has the ability to keep us dying for a long time, and with encouragement from family and friends, we may agree to treatments that lead only to needless suffering.

Hattie Bryant

One woman told me this tragic story about her brother-in-law whose heart stopped. When his family found him, his brain had been without oxygen for ten minutes. He was rushed to an ER, where he was resuscitated and his body temperature lowered. The man's cardiologist recommended against the body cooling and the waiting for twenty-four hours, as he believed that severe damage had been done already. It was the hospitalist, however, who didn't know the brother-in-law or what he would have wanted and who insisted standard protocols must be followed to see how the patient might fare.

Physicians do not have to live with what they do to us. Today, this gentleman is in a care facility while his wife tries to figure out how to pay for twenty-four-hour care, perhaps for decades. This man had an advance care plan, but decisions were made which got him exactly what he never wanted. This once vital sixty-five-year-old man will live out the remainder of his days with the mind of a five-year-old, the result of the damage his brain sustained due to loss of oxygen.

Palliative care physicians have taught me that our physical symptoms in the dying process can be relieved. It is our stubborn resistance to the death of our body that causes suffering. The agnostic physicians and nurses I know call this existential angst. We believers who resist need that famous prayer, "I do believe; help me overcome my unbelief!" (Mark 9:24, NIV). Resistance to death will bring suffering. Resistance—in the form of more procedures, more medicine, and more technologies—can rob us of the experience of seeing our loved ones who have gone before us come to get us. Resistance can prevent us from engaging with our loved ones here. Resistance can prevent us from listening to our favorite songs or talking with God.

Preparing the Ones We Love

The life of Jesus is exemplary in so many ways, and perhaps nowhere so clearly as when he teaches us how to kindly instruct those who love us when it is our time to die. He gives us our template: We are to talk. We are to communicate our deepest desires to everyone we know and love.

In the run up to Jesus' death, he started telling his disciples what their future was going to be. They were confused and didn't understand what he was saying. Just as we give some grace to these men, we must give grace to our family and friends as well. They can't truly understand where we are and what we may want, but that doesn't mean we give in to them.

The disciples had spent three years following Jesus. He was the center of their lives. They loved him and couldn't see what their lives would be without him, let alone imagine going back to the lives they had before he called them to himself. They were not ready to let him go. Most of the people in your life will not be ready to let you go.

Unlike Jesus, we don't know when we will die; we only know that for sure it will happen. Jesus knew the trajectory of his death and out of his love for those who loved him, was trying very hard to tell his inner circle that he would die soon. Six days before his now-famous Last Supper with the disciples, Mary, the sister of Lazarus, did something extraordinary. She chose to pour very expensive perfume on Jesus' feet, then wipe it with her hair. Those observing her actions criticized her because in their view, she could have sold this highly valued liquid and used the money to feed the poor. Four days later, another woman pours precious perfume on Jesus' head, and the same complaints are voiced. In both instances, Jesus tells the disciples that the expensive perfume is symbolic for his burial that will happen soon, and reminds them presciently, "The poor will always be with you, but you will not always have me" (John 12:6–7, ICB). Jesus praised both women, and knowingly predicted that their act of compassion would be told about throughout history and to the world. These are beautiful examples from Jesus of why we want people with these women's compassion, selflessness, and understanding around when we are frail and seriously ill—people who simply wanted to be with Jesus as he was and to make him as comfortable as they knew how to do.

Jesus said to his disciples, "Do not let your hearts be troubled.[54] My appointed time is near.[55] I will die as the Scriptures say I will[56] and I will be seated at the right hand of the mighty God.[57] I confer on you my kingdom[58] and after I go and prepare a place for you, I will come back and take you to myself.[59] I won't leave you as orphans. I will come back to you.[60] As the Father has loved me so have I loved you,[61] so love each other as I have loved you.[62] Greater love has no man than to lay down his life for his friends."[63]

Defining Friends and "Family"

Jesus' mother never dreamed that she would watch her son die. We all know that children are supposed to bury their parents, not the other way around. He was probably thirty-three years old, and we have no record of him ever being physically ill or having any physical aches and pains, except for the hunger from his forty-day fast. We do know he was often heartsick over us. He wept and was sad because he knew the untapped glorious potential of every soul and wanted us to have what he had planned for us. He was probably disappointed when his own family told others that they thought he was crazy (Mark 3:20–21). His own family had a hard time believing

54 John 14:1
55 Matthew 26:18
56 Mark 14:21
57 Luke 22:69
58 Luke 22:29
59 John 14:3
60 John 14:18
61 John 15:9
62 John 15:12
63 John 15:14

he was who he claimed to be. In typical Jesus fashion, he does the unexpected and surprises everyone by giving "family" an entirely new definition!

> Then His mother and His brothers arrived, and standing outside they sent word to Him and called Him. A crowd was sitting around Him, and they said to Him, "Behold, Your mother and Your brothers are outside looking for You." Answering them, He said, "Who are My mother and My brothers?" Looking about at those who were sitting around Him, He said, "Behold You are My mother and My brothers! For whoever does the will of God, he is My brother and sister and mother." (Mark 3:31–35, NASB)

This is significant for a couple of reasons. Family, and especially in those days, was extremely important. It defined your history, your status and even your future. Jesus understood that, but he also knew who he was beyond the human persona he embodied. There was no one more important than the Father. It was the whole purpose of his ministry on earth, and what would ultimately cost him his life—and give us ours. Second, he understood family dynamics far better than we ever will, but rather than turning his back on his immediate family, he was sending the signal that they—and we—are part of a much bigger family to whom we can and should turn for support.

He affirms this belief from the cross as Jesus remembers his mother, aching for her and all of us as he looks at her and at his beloved disciple, John. "When Jesus saw his mother and his favorite disciple with her, he said to his mother, 'This man is now your son.' Then to the disciple, 'She is now your mother'" (John 19:26–27, CEV).

Hope for the Best, Plan for the Worst

It is not uncommon for the family whom you trust and expect the most from to have the most difficulty following through on your wishes for your end-of-life care. Some will tell your doctors that you are crazy or not thinking straight. The rich and famous have splashed these stories all over the newspapers. It is a burden to be so wealthy that many fight over your money. Tom Benson, the owner of the New Orleans Saints, made some changes to his business structure; his daughter took him to court, arguing that he had lost his mind. She lost. It's even more dramatic when your ability to think is in dispute, and you are not able to fight back as Tom Benson did.

If you're old enough, you may remember "Top-40" radio legend Casey Kasem, whose own final days might make somebody's Top-40 worst-deaths list. Casey had grown children by his first wife. From 1980 onward he was married to another woman who, according to reports, never embraced his children. When he was too sick to speak for himself due to advanced Lewy body dementia, his daughter and wife fought over his end-of-life care. Mr. Kasem had given them *both* durable power of attorney for healthcare—and thus a multi-decade emotional pot was stirred when the daughter disagreed with the wife. The big public brawl over Mr. Kasem's end-of-life care is an example of the problems that can occur when we do not provide clear instructions for family, friends, and physicians.

Don't Leave Your Dying to Others

The Patient Self Determination Act (PSDA) passed by Congress in 1990 made it illegal for clinicians to do anything to you without your permission. This means that doctors cannot and will not make end-of-life care decisions for you. This seems only right—except for the unanticipated reality that occurs when we fail to make our end-of-life wishes known and communicated before we can no longer speak for ourselves. Legally and ethically, clinicians will do everything in their power to keep you alive through the power of modern medicine.

Experience shows that when your end is near, you will begin to lose an interest in things that used to interest you. Football scores, politics, favorite TV shows, reading, and the obituaries just won't be that important anymore. Your loved ones may realize that you aren't eating. They don't understand that food isn't all that important anymore either and that you just aren't hungry. Experience also tells us that invariably, someone in your family will insist that you eat. The person might even say, "Don't act so crazy," or "Stop being silly and just eat." They may even want to take you to the hospital, so that a feeding tube can be inserted to keep you nourished. Are you ready to face that possibility?

Creating Your Circle of Care

The rate of death by accident in the United States is just over 5 percent.[64] This means you are likely to live a fairly long life and that when death comes, it probably won't be immediate. Safe water, clean air, and a decent food supply also contribute to longer life expectancies in this country. And, of course, we have modern medicine with its massive amount of complex technologies and billions of dollars invested to keep us alive. These are the very reasons you need a Circle of Care.

Just like you took personal responsibility for other major decisions in your life, you are ultimately responsible for your healthcare and end-of-life treatment decisions. Remember that being the decision-maker doesn't mean you are alone in and through the process. It means that the thinking starts with you, and the pages provided in this study will walk you through the steps designed to help you to understand your options, document your choices, and communicate those choices to those most important to you in your life: family, friends, physician, neighbors, clergy, attorney, etc.

---

64 Hannah Nichols, "The top 10 leading causes of death in the United States," February 23, 2017, accessed November 28, 2018, https://www.medicalnewstoday.com/articles/282929.php

Hattie Bryant

More specifically, you will have the opportunity to decide to name a person and a backup, known as your healthcare proxy (or proxy, surrogate, durable power of attorney for healthcare, agent, or decision-maker), who will be the one person who will represent you and your wishes if you lose the ability to make complex decisions. This is not the same as your durable power of attorney, who would be responsible for your assets. It is probably best that your healthcare proxy is not the same person as your durable power of attorney. Using the tools in the workbook, and sharing your decisions with everyone you know and love, is the greatest gift that you can give yourself and your Circle of Care.

Death without Fear in the Modern Age

My girlfriend Lyle gave me permission to share about her mom's sweet death:

> My mom, Lynn Holland, came to Christ when I was a teenager. She sought God, found God, knew God, got close to God. She talked about heaven a lot. She told me and my brother, Peter, that she was very ready to go to heaven and she said this more than once—it was a theme of her life as she aged. She said, "I can't wait to get to heaven," and it wasn't because she complained of a hard life here; she was just ready to move on. There was a peace about her—she was happy where the Lord had her. She was a caregiver, she saw a lot of death and she was not afraid of it at all which for me was the greatest gift. She taught my brother and I not to be afraid, and for her to talk about death didn't seem unusual to us.
>
> Mom was 79, taking no medication, fit and active when she started complaining of a sore foot and thought she had gout. It was only when she went to the hospital to have it checked out that we learned she had dropped a jar on her foot.
>
> When I called the hospital I was told she had gone for an MRI and to please call back in about one hour. Before I called back her best friend called to say that she thought Mom had had a cardiac arrest. I quickly was able to talk with her ER doctor. He was the physician on duty when the code for her resuscitation came in. He explained that prior to the MRI she was given a heavy dose of a pain medication and while in the MRI her heart had stopped for twenty minutes. He said he was able get her heart going again and he had cooled her body to help prevent cell damage. He said, "We won't know what's going on with her for 24 hours."
>
> I prayed, "Lord, is she gone?" And, he said "yes." I knew. I knew. When your heart stops for twenty minutes your brain is affected. I knew when the doctor was talking that this was bad. I told my husband, "She's gone and I have to get there."

I flew to Phoenix the next day to find my brother at the hospital sitting with her. I saw her but I knew it wasn't my mother. I opened her eyelid and looked in and knew she wasn't there. This was just her body. When I finally accepted that she was with God my heart flooded with joy and happiness as I knew the reward we are promised was finally hers. I was overwhelmed that God had been so gracious to her to just put her to sleep and carry her home.

We met with the neurologist and he told us what was going on physically. He said, "She is not technically brain-dead as her brain stem—in the neck—is still alive. The tissue in her cranium is dead. There is no activity up there but her stem is still active. She won't be able to think, feel, move, talk—she is comatose. The person you know is not there." By modern medical standards she was still alive because ICU technologies made it so.

Mom had it right about what it means to be a Christian. It is knowing that you are going to live with God. This life on earth is not the end, it is just a part of our journey.

My brother and I didn't even have to look at each other. We just said, "Unhook her."

Lynn Holland gave her children a worship experience right there in the ICU. She was not afraid to die, and not afraid to talk about it. As a result, her children were not afraid for her or for themselves.

A Foretaste of Forever

"He will wipe away every tear from their eyes. There will be no more death or mourning or crying or pain, for the old order of things has passed away . . . 'I am making everything new!'" (Revelation 21:4–5, NIV).

God hasn't called me out yet so I sit here and write, praying that he will use these words to give you what he has given me—a yearning to see him face to face. "Oh that will be glory for me, when by his grace I shall look on his face."

When all my labors and trials are o'er,
And I am safe on that beautiful shore,
Just to be near the dear Lord I adore,
Will through the ages be glory for me.

Oh, that will be glory for me,
Glory for me, glory for me,

Hattie Bryant

When by His grace I shall look on His face,
That will be glory, be glory for me.

When, by the gift of His infinite grace,
I am accorded in heaven a place,
Just to be there and to look on His face,
Will through the ages be glory for me.

Friends will be there I have loved long ago;
Joy like a river around me will flow;
Yet just a smile from my Savior, I know,
Will through the ages be glory for me.[65]

   To gain an even greater sense of that tomorrow, listen to David Phelps sing "Heaven's Shore"[66]—and then try to convince yourself that it's better here than there.

65 Charles H. Gabriel, "Oh, That Will Be Glory" (1900). Public domain.
66 David Phelps, "Heaven's Shore (Live)," YouTube video, September 11, 2015, https://www.youtube.com/watch?v=Jr34087qHcl (accessed June 16, 2018).

Choose a Proxy and Provide Specific Instructions

Big Word for This Session: COMMUNITY

Share each other's burdens,
and in this way obey the law of Christ.
— GALATIANS 6:2, NLT

Opening

Optional Listening: "Give Me Jesus," found at illhaveitgodsway.com/biblestudy
Opening Prayer: Father God, show us fresh insight now, as we open ourselves to you. We ask this humbly in the name of Jesus, Amen.

Take some time to discuss the homework. Was there anything in the questions or readings that was especially interesting or impactful?

 ## Play the Session Four video.

Available on the DVD or from the link found on this page: illhaveitgodsway.com/biblestudy

Video Discussion

1. What is the Patient Self-Determination Act? How does this change the way we communicate with physicians?

2. What are the problems that can arise if you choose a spouse or a child for a proxy?

3. Is choosing a proxy *enough*? Explain.

4. Why does everybody "need a Hattie"?

Memorize this:

Doctors do not make end-of-life decisions. You do. Since most of us will be too weak toward the end of this life to sort out complex medical choices, we need a proxy. You must define what is important to you and you must speak. Express yourself—come clean! Create a Circle of Care starting with selecting a proxy and a backup.

Hattie Bryant

Think about people you know who . . .
- Would be willing to speak for you.
- Can separate their personal desires for you from *your* desires for you.
- Would take some time soon to review with you what you are writing in this document.
- Live close to you; can travel to you quickly; or work via phone, email, and text with a physician.
- Are young enough and healthy enough to be around in the future.
- You trust with your life.
- Can calmly manage any conflicts.
- Can stand up to family members who may not agree with you.
- Can negotiate with physicians to achieve your stated goals and be willing to fire a physician who doesn't listen.
- Can listen to facts presented and make a rational decision.

As people come to mind, list them in the Circle of Care worksheet on page 109.

5. What problems can arise if you choose someone who is afraid of death for you—or for themselves?

The best way to help your proxy is to tell everyone in your Circle of Care who that proxy is and who the backup proxy is and give everyone the same information you have given your proxies.

6. Read Mark 3:31–35 and John 19:26–27. How did Jesus redefine family? Even so, what did Jesus do for his mother?

7. Read Mark 8:31–38 and John 12:6–7. How did Jesus prepare his own Circle of Care for his death?

8. Recall Lyle's story on pages 101–102. What did Lyle's mom do for her children?

9. Why do you think pastors punt on dealing with death in advance?

10. Does your local church/parish help members face death with joy? Does it help members make a worship experience out of death? If not, how can you be part of making that happen?

11. How might you start a small group or ministry around spiritual formation that prepares us to die, so we can really live?

12. How might asking your neighbors to be in your Circle of Care impact them?

Closing Prayer:

Father, help us see what you want us to see. Dispel any fears or anxieties we have about our own death and the death of those we love. Set us free! In Christ's name we ask, Amen.

Before the next group session, complete the following homework. There is no reading assignment this week.

Hattie Bryant

MY CIRCLE OF CARE

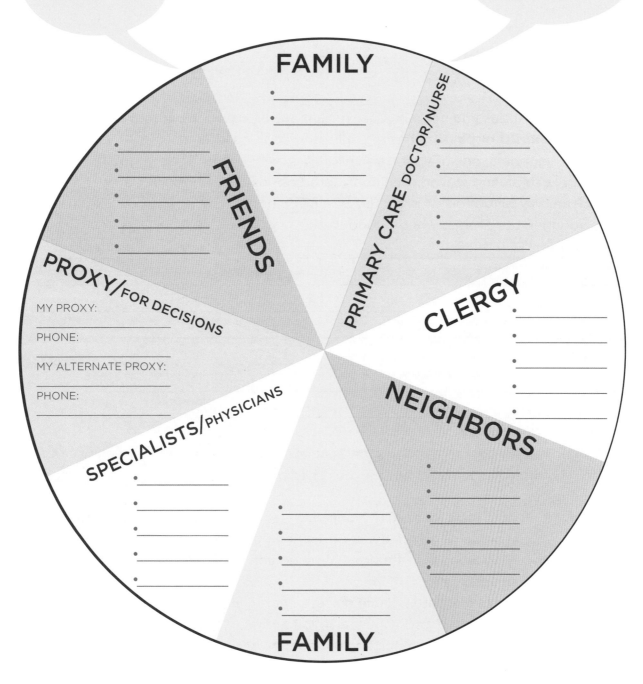

Add names to each section of your Circle of Care!

Transfer the names in your finalized Circle of Care to pages 150 and 157.

FAMILY

PRIMARY CARE DOCTOR/NURSE

FRIENDS

CLERGY

PROXY/FOR DECISIONS

MY PROXY:

PHONE:

MY ALTERNATE PROXY:

PHONE:

NEIGHBORS

SPECIALISTS/PHYSICIANS

FAMILY

HOMEWORK

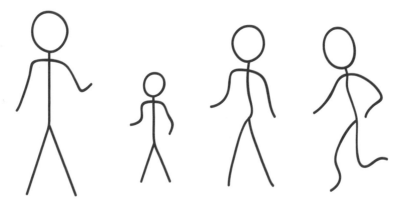

Review the qualities you need in a proxy that are listed on the top of page 107 and write your list of possibilities e.g. minister; adult children of your friends; nieces; nephews; neighbors; one of your own children—the one who is feisty, outspoken, strong, persistent, and maybe even considered obnoxious; a godchild; a cousin; a sibling—much younger one; the spouse of a niece or nephew; or your own spouse—if much younger, but probably not a good choice:

1._____

2._____

3._____

4._____

5._____

6._____

7._____

Remember: It's best to name one person, not a committee. There are plenty of reasons that this person might not be your child or your spouse. At the same time, it is your choice.

We don't want to leave our proxy alone. We want a Circle of Care that is ready, willing, and able to help us go gently to God when the time comes. Too many Americans are dying alone in institutions. Why do you think this is happening? (Too many broken relationships.)

Now is the time to cultivate a Circle of Care—not when you get sick or become frail. Do this now. There is a good chance, if you are in a group study with this book, that you have figured out the importance of community.

We must also prepare spiritually. In Reading 3, you read my go-to-for-strength verses. Please look up each of these verses, take a few minutes to meditate on each one, then write your own translation. Be prepared to read some of these passages aloud in your group next week. And, add your own verses to share. Just think of what you can do as a group to enlarge this list!

Exodus 14:14

Deuteronomy 31:8

Psalm 23

Psalm 25:8–10

Psalm 34:4

Psalm 46:10

Psalm 55:22

Psalm 61:2–3

Psalm 73:23–26

Psalm 91:14–16

Isaiah 41:10

Jeremiah 29:11

Matthew 28:11

2 Corinthians 4:6

1 John 3:1

1 John 4:4

Revelation 21:4

SPIRITUAL ASSESSMENT

Your doctor(s) are part—just part—of your Circle of Care. They are encouraged to ask you for a "spiritual assessment." Most don't! There are many of these tools available for doctors, but most don't take the time to think about this topic.

Surprise your doctor by giving him or her your spiritual assessment. You don't have to wait for them to ask you to answer these questions; most specialists won't bother, and even your primary care doctor might not want to take the time to ask you these questions. The answers to these questions will change the course of your discussion, as you are making it very clear that while you have a normal fear of death, it is being managed with the spiritual tools you have been putting in place for decades (or maybe just since you started this study).

Print this out, fill in your answers and take it to your next doctor appointment.

H.O.P.E.[67]

H: Sources of hope	What are your sources of hope, strength, comfort, and peace?
	What do you hold on to during difficult times?
O: Organized religion	Are you part of a religious or spiritual community?
	Does it help you? How?
P: Personal spirituality and practices	Do you have personal spiritual beliefs?
	What aspects of your spirituality or spiritual practices do you find most helpful?
E: Effects on medical care and end-of-life issues	Does your current situation affect your ability to do the things that usually help you spiritually?
	As a doctor, is there anything that I can do to help you access the resources that usually help you?
	Are there any specific practices or restrictions I should know about in providing your medical care?
	If the patient is dying: How do your beliefs affect the kind of medical care you would like me to provide over the next few days/weeks/months?

---

67 G. Anandarajah and E. Hight, "Spirituality and Medical Practice: Using the HOPE Questions as a Practical Tool for Spiritual Assessment," *American Family Physician.* 63, no. 1 (2001): 87, accessed June 16, 2018, https://www.aafp.org/afp/2001/0101/p81.html. Adapted with permission.

There is no reading assignment, as we'll save Reading 5 as our last reading for our closing session in this study.

If you like, you can look at the video to be presented in the next session. It is full of information that may be new, and you may want to watch it more than once. You can also review this session video at illhaveitgodsway.com/biblestudy.

Create the
Best Gift Ever

Big Word for This Session: COMMUNICATE

Finally, let the mighty strength of the Lord make you strong.
— EPHESIANS 6:10, CEV

Opening

Optional Listening: "Heaven's Shore," found at illhaveitgodsway.com/biblestudy
Opening Prayer: Father God, show us fresh insight now, as we open ourselves to you. We ask this humbly in the name of Jesus, Amen.

Take some time to discuss the homework. Was there anything in the questions or readings that was especially interesting or impactful? Did everyone make a list on page 110?

Let's get some answers to questions we still might have before you put your plan in writing and get ready to share it with your Circle of Care.

 Play the Session Five video.
Available on the DVD or from the link found on this page:
illhaveitgodsway.com/biblestudy

Video Discussion

1. Have you been around family members or friends who have lost decisional capacity?

2. Have you seen family members convince the seriously ill to take aggressive treatments or take over a seriously ill or frail person's life?

3. How does a doctor determine that you have decisional capacity?

4. Are there times when we might not want everything modern medicine has to offer? How will you know when to say no?

5. Have you known people who didn't know when to say no?

6. How do we make it easy for a proxy to do his or her job for us?

I talk in the video about page 206 in your workbook—my other book, *I'll Have It My Way*. You did this same exercise in this study on page 61.

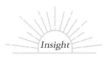 Medicine cannot give us what we need for a peaceful death. It can deal with physical pain but not spiritual or emotional pain. We have to get ourselves ready and we can't wait until we become frail or seriously ill.

The MOST IMPORTANT few minutes of our entire study are upon us.

To create the best gift ever to give to your Circle of Care, copy the names from page 109 to pages 150 and 157; copy your choice from page 61 to page 150; copy your choices from page 88 to page 151; copy what you wrote from page 89 to page 152; and, from your list of potential proxies on page 110, choose your proxy and a backup. Add those names to page 153. Since we've already done the thinking and writing, this should not take much time.

We will serve as each other's witnesses to create legal documents now.

 ## Play the video of Hattie's Simple Directive.
Available on the DVD or from the link found on this page:
illhaveitgodsway.com/biblestudy

Here's an example of a little script idea.

Hi Everyone. You can see that this is Hattie talking. I want you to know that today I have completed an advance care directive that is different from other types of documents. I have named my healthcare proxy and her name is Falyn Curtis. I have given to Falyn and many others specific instructions if there comes a time when I won't be able to speak with physicians on my own behalf. I want you to know that I am not afraid to die, and that I am actually looking forward to heaven. Don't be afraid for me or yourselves! There are a few things that are important to me that I want to be able to do until I die. For example, I want to be able to chew and swallow. And I mean chew! I don't want to live on liquids. I want to be able to engage with others, I want to be able to breathe on my own; I want to be able to toilet myself. There's more on my list, but you get the idea. **If the time comes that I am not able to do any of these things, do not call 911, call Falyn who in turn will engage hospice care. I insist: DNH, do not hospitalize and DNR—do not resuscitate! Thank you all for being such a sweet part of my life.**

I just recorded this, and it took seventy-two seconds. Personalize this, and just do it!

In my book *I'll Have It My Way*, there is an extensive glossary of medical terms which includes DNH, or Do Not Hospitalize. This term gets a great deal of attention when I speak, which is why I am pointing it out to you specifically here. When you read my directive in essay form, which you can find on pages 140–142, I am clearly demanding DNH when I am no longer able to do the things that are important to me. DNH does not mean do not treat. It means do not dial 911 and only comfort care or palliative care is to be provided in my home. No one ever is required to go to a hospital. It's your choice.

Make Your Own Video!

Now, before we finish today, everyone take out your cell phones and find the video mode in your camera. Trade phones with a partner, and go ahead and put on video what you've just written. (Those who have phones: Please volunteer to record your friends who might not have a phone.)

Again, this is the most important homework assignment of all.

Closing Prayer:

Father, help us see what you want us to see. Dispel any fears or anxieties we have about our own death and the death of those we love. Set us free! In Christ's name we ask, Amen.

Before the next group session, complete the following homework and Reading 5. This week's homework is an extension of the activities we did in today's session.

HOMEWORK

1. Make copies of pages 149–157 at the end of this book. Take them to the people in your Circle of Care.

2. Send your video to the Circle of Care and anyone else you want to include. Please help anyone in your group who does not have a phone with video functionality. Post it on your Facebook page. Why not? Don't forget to send it to your doctor. And please send it to Hattie@IllHaveItMyWay.com, and I'll post it along with mine.

    Next week, be prepared to share your experience with the group!

    Before the next session, be sure to complete Reading 5 on pages 121–128. You can also review the Session Five videos at illhaveitgodsway.com/biblestudy.

Start Living in God's Kingdom Now

Accept That We Are Not God and We Will All Die
Learn the Limits of Modern Medicine
Understand Our Healthcare Choices
Choose a Proxy and Provide Specific Instructions
Start Living in God's Kingdom Now

Create in me a clean heart oh God
and renew a right spirit within me.
— PSALM 51:10, KJV

The gospel is not just about being saved for eternity; it is about being saved to be fully alive in Christ now—and while we're at it, we are supposed to change the world! This has nothing to do with physicians or medicine. It's an inside job. It's God our Father, Jesus the Son, and the Holy Spirit in us, with us, and for us. It's surrendering our will to God's will. When we do this, we become like Jesus; we walk around as if Jesus is living our life for us. We are the light of the world. We are the salt. We don't have to wait for our bodies to quit to be alive in and with Christ. We can live the words of the prayer we've known since childhood: "Your kingdom come, your will be done *on earth* as it is in heaven."

Sadly, and counter to God's desire for us, we live our lives exemplifying Henry David Thoreau's assessment: "The mass of men lead lives of quiet desperation." Why are so many of us Christians missing the Kingdom of God at work right now, in this world and in our lives?

We Reap What We Sow

Over the years of my research on this topic, many clinicians have told me that people die the way they lived. It makes sense. As long as we are living with fear, anger, envy, bitterness, worry, regret, remorse, pride, and our it's all-about-me adolescent demands, then when we do become frail or hear a serious diagnosis, we become more fearful, more angry, more bitter, more worried, more full of regret, more remorseful, more demanding, and more selfish. Under stress we default to our defaults—and for sure, hearing that we have a life-limiting illness is stressful.

None of my sitting in church for sixty-plus years got my attention more than learning this from veteran clinicians when I suffered a massive heart attack. No, it wasn't one that required a physician or anything modern medicine had to offer; this was the other kind of broken heart.

I decided I must have been the cause of what happened. Luke 6:43–45 comes to mind: "A good person brings good things out of the good stored up in his heart, and an evil person brings things out of the evil stored up in his heart. For the mouth speaks what the heart is full of" (Luke 6:45, NIV). I must be angry or judgmental or something terrible, or this would not have happened, so I asked God to give me a heart transplant. Then I remembered the words David had prayed, "Create in me a clean heart, O God, and renew a right spirit within me" (Psalm 51:10, KJV). So I stopped asking for a new heart and starting asking for a pure heart—a clean heart, a right heart.

> Hear my cry, O God, listen to my prayer; from the end of the earth I call to you when my heart is faint. Lead me to the rock that is higher than I, for you have been my refuge, a strong tower against the enemy. (Psalm 61:1–3, ESV)

I also realized that God would be there to help, but I had to do a lot of the work myself. He taught me that there is no room for what he has for me if I'm full of what I think works. So I embarked on a journey to rid my heart of the wrong things and replace them with the right things:

Hearts stuffed with too many wrong things . . .	Hearts full of a few right things . . .
self-absorbed, selfish, arrogant, hostile, acrimony, detesting, despising, disgusted, hateful, loathsome, malicious, repelled, spiteful, resentful	**LOVE**
anguishing, ungrateful, entitled, desolate, blue, sad, agonizing, disheartened, cynical, jealous, miserable, gloomy, melancholy, depressed, neurotic, despairing	**JOY**
uncertain, concerned, angry, edgy, nervous, troubled, apprehensive, noisy, fearful, shocked, vexed, desperate, distressed, upset, tense, doubtful, restless, worried, irascible, distracted, at war, in chaos, jumpy, strained, stressed, despairing, agitated, anxious	**PEACE**

impertinent, impulsive, nervous, scared, contrarian, willful, exasperated, defiant, irritated, petulant, resentful, anxious, peevish, offended, disobedient, fretful	**PATIENCE**
spiteful, grim, acerbic, nitpicky, cruel, critical, brutish, callous, churlish, virulent, disinterested, hateful, back biting, inconsiderate, insensitive, malevolent, ruthless, savage, thoughtless, severe, greedy, hard-hearted, vitriolic, judgmental, brutal, cold-blooded, harsh, selfish, tough, merciless, inhumane, mean	**KINDNESS**
bad, corrupt, crooked, depraved, dishonest, evil, evildoing, indecent, low, fault-finding, liar, gossip, improper, underhanded, vile, wicked, indiscrete, perverted, unscrupulous, immoral	**GOODNESS**
weak, wishy-washy, uncertain, undependable, flaky, fickle, false, shaky, slack, inconstant, untrue, slipshod, wavering, vacillating, untrustworthy, two-timing, traitor, disloyal, cheater, capricious, corrupt, perfidious, recreant, deceitful	**FAITHFULNESS**
abrasive, severe, harsh, loud, demanding, aggressive, abrupt, cruel, hard, stern	**GENTLENESS**
gluttonous, blunt, pleasure-seeking, greedy, unrestrained, thrill-seeking, overindulgent, weak, frail, feeble, uninhibited, indulgent, slothful, wild, wanton, decadent, lazy	**SELF-CONTROL**

We can spend the rest of our years on earth taking the default position, due to our poor habits—or we can schedule our heart surgery with God today, and watch the impossible unfold.

Designing Life from the Inside Out

Interior designer and author, Leah RIchardson, speaks often to Christian women and she tells how she starts on a renovation project. She sweetly removes excess piles of stuff from her client's home. If she had her way, she would remove much more than the client is willing to give up. Just like our closets and garages, our heart can be loaded with the useless and the damaging. What we carry around in there can kill us.

Fear, anger (especially as it morphs into contempt), envy, bitterness, worry, regret, remorse, and pride do kill. These emotions are sin, and no amount of sanitizing these words in psychology and therapeutic language changes this fact. The reality is that these emotions give us hard hearts packed hard and tight, with little room for God to move. Women complain a lot about emotionally unavailable men, but in my own life I had become emotionally unavailable to God. I was too busy trying to be what I thought he wanted me to be, and wasted a lot of life until I learned he doesn't care about what I do, or what I accomplish. He cares about my heart. It's the old Mary-Martha battle. These are the sisters you can read about in Luke 10:38–42. Martha was busy preparing a meal, while Mary sat at the feet of Jesus. Many of us are good at being Martha and others are good at being Mary. We want to be good at being both.

I have friends who make a living as psychologists and therapists. I respect and admire them, have benefited from their deep insights and guidance, and have learned by reading books they have assigned. I know that they have many clients who are not Christians who get the same insights and guidance and read the same books and manage to get through their deep struggles without God. Does that mean that God isn't really necessary in times of trouble? To the contrary, "God is patient, because he wants everyone to turn from sin and no one to be lost" (2 Peter 3:9, CEV). The difference is that as a believer, I don't want us to just *get through*. I want to thrive and enjoy God's kingdom now.

Open Heart Surgery

Living in God's Kingdom now means you might need heart surgery or a total transplant; and like any serious operation, it takes time and preparation. This is about character formation. It is about having the mind of Christ and the heart of God. And specifically, it is about letting go of your will to live and to work on God's ideas, not yours. I have been making a living talking to businesspeople about business since 1979, and now God has me talking about the topic nobody wants to talk about. You would think doctors would find it easy to tell patients the truth—you are dying—but no, they'll think of anything else to talk about, especially how medicine can keep you going—just not the truth. You would think pastors would find it easy to talk about death to comfort the dying and their loved ones, but no. One pastor told me, "The church punts on everything, including death and dying." Until God tells me otherwise, I'll pick up my cross and keep walking and talking.

You have individual talents and abilities, dreams and plans. At the same time, God is more interested in your character than in your accomplishing anything or taking any specific action. While I used to be very good at making my to-do list, now I ask God to give me *his* to-do list. My husband Bruce asks God for his marching orders before he gets out of bed, and most often Bruce hears from God in his sleep. That doesn't happen for me.

How do we get out of ourselves? How do we die to self? Do we have to leave everything we know and love to escape our small, silly selves? Leaving your old self behind doesn't mean you have to give up your hairdresser, your grocery store, or your favorite jeans. What it does mean is that we have to get our hearts right, so that without thinking we make the right choices, say the right things, and do the things God has got for us to do. The Great Physician has been into making hearts new since that apple-eating incident. He promised the Israelites more than once that if they will come back to him, he will fix their hearts.

The Bible does not shrink from graphic descriptions, but as Dr. Peter Kreeft writes, "God is not a pop psychologist; God is a warrior."[68] A cozy conversation with Oprah won't get us what we need. We need our warrior God to cut out of us the sins—thoughts and feelings—that weigh us down and keep us from God's healing.

God, your God, will cut away the thick calluses on your heart and your children's hearts, freeing you to love God, Your God, with your whole heart and soul and live, really live. (Deuteronomy 30:6, MSG)

I will give you a new heart and put a new spirit in you; I will remove from you your heart of stone and give you a heart of flesh. (Ezekiel 36:26, NIV)

Our heart is restless until it rests in you. — Augustine[69]

Pure hearts are living in God's Kingdom now because their heart shows them God. If our hearts aren't right we don't see God, and we don't see the Kingdom of God in our home, our neighborhood, our church, our friends.

Open the eyes of their hearts, and let the light of your truth flood in. Shine Your light on the hope you are calling them to embrace. (Ephesians 1:18, VOICE)

The Heart Sees All

Ephesians 4:18–19 (NIV) explains why we can't see the Kingdom of God right now: "They are darkened in their understanding and separated from the life of God

---

68 Kreeft, *I Burned for Your Peace*, 233.
69 Saint Augustine, *Confessions* (Oxford: Oxford University Press, 2008), 3.

because of the ignorance that is in them due to the hardening of their hearts. Having lost all sensitivity, they have given themselves over to _____" (fill in the blank). Consider that you, like me, have given yourself over to fear, anger, envy, bitterness, worry, regret, remorse, pride, and selfish demands.

Jesus came to set us free from these heart-hardening emotions. He did this by eliminating rules and death and by replacing them with love and life. Jesus wants to give us what Dallas Willard calls "The Kingdom Heart."[70] It's this Kingdom Heart that sees heaven now. It's this Kingdom Heart that sees death as the door to our real home, and getting this new heart means our inner self has to change. Dr. Willard also quotes Matthew 6:21, where Jesus says, "Your heart will be where your treasure is." He goes on to say, "Remember that our heart is our will, or our spirit: the center of our being from which our life flows. It is what gives orientation to everything we do. A heart rightly directed therefore brings health and wholeness to the entire personality."[71]

Feeding Our Spirit

In addition to health and wholesomeness, God bestows upon the healthy heart certain rights and benefits that are ours to embrace and enjoy. They are beautifully captured in the Psalms, where King David, a man after God's own heart, and its other writers poured out their joyful, fearful, and broken hearts to God.

> **I can be bold:** "Test me, LORD, and try me, examine my heart and my mind" (Psalm 26:2, NIV).
> **I can confess and praise:** "My flesh and my heart may fail, but God is the strength of my heart and my portion forever" (Psalm 73:26, NIV).
> **Like David begging after being called out for murder and adultery I can, no matter what I've done, throw myself on God's mercy:** "Create in me a pure heart, O God, and renew a steadfast spirit within me" (Psalm 51:10, NIV).
> **I can take instruction:** "Take delight in the LORD, and he will give you the desires of your heart" (Psalm 37:4, NIV); "The one who has clean hands and a pure heart, who does not trust in an idol or swear by a false god" (Psalm 24:4, NIV).
> **I can praise God:** "I will give thanks to you, LORD, with all my heart; I will tell of all your wonderful deeds" (Psalm 9:1, NIV).
> **I can ask for consideration:** "May these words of my mouth and this meditation of my heart be pleasing in your sight, LORD, my Rock and my Redeemer" (Psalm 19:14, NIV).

---

70 Willard, *The Divine Conspiracy*, 129.
71 Ibid, 206.

Hattie Bryant

I can ask for direction: "I call as my heart grows faint; lead me to the rock that is higher than I" (Psalm 61:2, NIV).

Whatever the condition of your heart, spend some time in the Psalms. Pastor Rick Warren suggests an exercise for those of us who have hurting hearts: He suggests that as you read, mark in one color all of the Psalms you identify with, and in another color mark the ones that encourage you. You'll discover that others have been where you are—in highs and lows and everything in between—and that God has been there in each and every one.

As Goes the Heart

Broken hearts are better than hard hearts. I can tell you that a broken heart can mend correctly at the hand of the great surgeon and healer, Jesus. A pastor at the church I attended for many years delivered a line in a sermon that I will never forget, and have shared with many friends when they were hurting. He said, "No matter what things look like from the outside, life is fair. It breaks everybody's heart." In 2010, this pastor died at the age of eighty-two of complications from a heart attack.

Except for all the killings in wars, the number-one killer of human beings throughout the history of civilization is the heart stopping. The pump called your heart will stop one day, and between now and then you have millions of tiny decisions to make that will give you love and joy all the way to the last beat or will turn anger, fear, regret, remorse, envy, or any destructive thoughts or feelings into a deeply nuanced web of entanglements that prevents a peaceful passing over to perfection.

Two women my age have told me the same story about watching their moms die in the care of expert hospice teams. They both said they were not happy because no matter how much medication was brought to bear, their mothers were fretting and had anguish on their faces until their last breath. No amount of medicine can make up for a life filled with regrets, anger, and bitterness, and certainly won't give us what we need for a sweet, peaceful passing.

What benefits come to us when we let go of what we think works to make room for all the good that God's got for us? We get the Kingdom Heart now, and this heart doesn't lose a beat. This heart brings us into the presence of our King Jesus, face to face. As the old hymn says, "Oh that will be glory for me, when by his grace I will look on his face, that will be glory, be glory for me!" When you open the eyes of your heart to see the Kingdom come to earth as it is in heaven, you will see yourself resurrected up and out of the old small self and living large now into God's great plan.

> *God . . . has planted eternity in the human heart.*
> — Ecclesiastes 3:11, NLT

Start Living in God's Kingdom Now

Big Word for This Session: JOY

From now on, then, you must live the rest of our earthly lives
controlled by God's will and not by human desires.
— 1 PETER 4:2, GNT

Opening

Optional Listening: "Because He Lives," found at illhaveitgodsway.com/biblestudy

Opening Prayer: Father God, show us fresh insight now, as we open ourselves to you. We ask this humbly in the name of Jesus, Amen.

Play the opening video.

Available on the DVD or from the link found on this page: illhaveitgodsway.com/biblestudy

Homework Discussion

Take some time to review the homework.

- How did it go for you, as you gave out your "gift" to family and friends? Did you forward the video around to others, or post it to a social-media page? What reactions did you get?

- Did you fill in the H.O.P.E. assessment for your physician? Did anyone deliver it? Again, what reactions did you get?

Going Deeper

1. Had it ever occurred to you that you will die the way you have lived? How did you react when you first read that statement?

2. What can you do about this?

3. Have you spent a lot of time trying to change other people? How did that go?

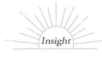

Insight

I am suggesting a massive heart change to get you back to your true self as God made you. It's not so much a getting of new self, as it is a letting go of what has been piled on you. How can we even breathe with all of this? Religious people tend to tweak around the edges, but that won't get us what God wants for us—true union with him.

4. Circle the words that you think describe what might be taking up space in your heart, and then share afterward.

FEAR ANGER CONTEMPT BITTERNESS WORRY PRIDE

ANXIETY REGRET REMORSE SELF-CENTEREDNESS ENVY JEALOUSY

5. What connection can you see between thoughts/emotions and behavior?

    Read aloud 2 Timothy 3:2–5.
    It's discouraging to read a list of all the ways we fall short. We are to "circumcise" our hearts. Deuteronomy 10:16 says:

    > Therefore, circumcise your heart and stop being stubborn. (ISV)
    > Therefore, cleanse your heart and stop being so stubborn! (NET)

    What does it mean to "stop being stubborn"? Our habits have piled up and calcified. Do you think you can fix yourself by yourself? Hold on:

    > And the Lord your God will circumcise our heart and the heart of your offspring, so that you will love the Lord your God with all your heart and with all your soul, that you may live. (Deuteronomy 30:6, ESV)

6. Read out loud: "Blessed are the pure in heart: for they shall see God" (Matthew 5:8, KJV). Does this verse scare you or inspire you? Why?

One dying woman told a nurse that she felt herself clearing out of the way, so God could fill her. Could we do this each morning as we wake? Yes, we could wake up praying, "Father, clear out my fears, worries, anxieties, negative thoughts about myself, and any emotion or word patterns that occupy my mind and heart—then come fill me with *you.*"

What Is a Kingdom Heart?

How do we get a Kingdom Heart? Fill up on God's healthy-heart diet! Stop asking yourself, "Can I have a Kingdom Heart? Can I be one with Christ? Really?" Read the following translations from 2 Peter:

He has by his own action given us everything that is necessary for living the truly good life, in allowing us to know the one who has called us to him, through his own glorious goodness. It is through him that God's greatest and most precious promises have become available to us men, making it possible for you to escape the inevitable disintegration that lust produced in the world and to share in God's essential nature. (2 Peter 1:3–4, PH)

Do you want more and more of God's kindness and peace? Then learn to know him better and better. For as you know him better, he will give you, through his great power, everything you need for living a truly good life: he even shares his own glory and his own goodness with us! And by that same mighty power he has given us all the other rich and wonderful blessings he promised; for instance, the promise to save us from the lust and rottenness all around us, and to give us his own character. (2 Peter 1:2–4, TLB)

May grace and peace be lavished on you as you grow in the rich knowledge of God and of Jesus our Lord!
I can pray this because his divine power has bestowed on us everything necessary for life and godliness through the rich knowledge of the one who called us by his own glory and excellence. Through these things he has bestowed on us his precious and most magnificent promises, so that by means of what was promised you may become partakers of the divine nature, after escaping the worldly corruption that is produced by evil desire. (2 Peter 1:2–4, NET)

Hattie Bryant

7. What does a heart-healthy diet look like?

How do we fill up with the right heart food? Step up to the banquet of Colossians 3:1–3, 9–14 (MSG):

> So, if you are serious about living this new resurrection life with Christ, act like it. Pursue the things over which Christ presides. Don't shuffle along, eyes to the ground, absorbed with the things right in front of you. Look up, and be alert to what is going on around Christ—that's where the action is. See things from *his* perspective.
>
> Your old life is dead. Your new life, which is your *real* life—is with Christ in God. *He* is your life. . . .
>
> You're done with that old life. It's like a filthy set of ill-fitting clothes you've stripped off and put in the fire. Now you're dressed in a new wardrobe. Every item of your new way of life is custom-made by the Creator, with his label on it. All the old fashions are now obsolete. Words like Jewish and non-Jewish, religious and irreligious, insider and outside, uncivilized and uncouth, slave and free, mean nothing. From now on everyone is defined by Christ, everyone is included in Christ.
>
> So, chosen by God for this new life of love, dress in the wardrobe God picked out for you: compassion, kindness, humility, quiet strength, discipline. Be even-tempered, content with second place, quick to forgive an offense. Forgive as quickly and completely as the Master forgave you.
>
> And regardless of what else you put on, wear love. It's your basic, all-purpose garment. Never be without it.

Your heart-healthy diet includes God's Word, prayer, worship, and service to others. This is simple, but not easy and not new. (Sorry.)

> Love the Lord your God with all your heart and with all your soul and with all your mind. This is the first and greatest commandment. (Matthew 22:37–38, NIV)

Here's what we do have to do to live in God's kingdom now:

1. Get on and stay on a spiritual growth path. Set aside time for meditation, prayer, fasting, study, worship. Live a life of simplicity, submission, service, and celebration. My favorite book for this is Richard Foster's *Celebration of Discipline*.

2. Surround yourself with others who do this, too.

3. Stop fretting so much over your body, your face, your hair . . . and get the best facelift from your own smile. Drop ten years (and a few pounds) just by standing up straight.

4. Move to improve.

5. Don't get sick, don't think about getting sick, and don't hang around people who are sick or who like to be sick (unless you are a volunteer in a caregiving situation or a family caregiver).

6. Stay social. Add to your circle of friends and your Circle of Care, and volunteer to be in someone else's circle.

7. Let your heart shine through your eyes.

8. Look for God in everyone and everything.

9. Stand up, throw your shoulders back, glance up to heaven, and put a smile on your face as you start your day thanking your Father that his kingdom is here now in what you are doing together.

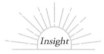 Live fully now, with heart, mind, body, and soul, all the way, every day in heaven on earth as we watch and are ever-ready to see Jesus face to face—to be done with what hurts, to embrace our perfect healing and wholeness.

 Play the closing video.
Available on the DVD or from the link found on this page: illhaveitgodsway.com/biblestudy

Closing Prayer:

Thank you, Father, for freeing us from fear we may have had about our own death and the death of those we love. Thank you for setting us free to live in your kingdom now, and until you call us home. In Christ's name we rejoice, Amen.

Complete the study on your own with the last few pages of homework.

HOMEWORK

Just because you've finished your study doesn't mean there isn't more to learn! Take some more time now, and work through the exercises that follow.

Write your own translations of these verses:

GOD, your God, will cut away the thick calluses on your heart and your children's hearts, freeing you to love GOD, Your God, with your whole heart and soul and live, really live. (Deuteronomy 30:6, MSG)

I'll give you a new heart. I'll put a new spirit in you. I'll cut out your stone heart and replace it with a red-blooded, firm muscled heart. Then you'll obey my statutes and be careful to obey my commands. You'll be my people! I'll be your God! (Ezekiel 11:19, MSG)

I will give you a new heart and put a new spirit in you; I will remove from you your heart of stone and give you a heart of flesh. (Ezekiel 36:26, NIV)

Your kingdom come, your will be done on earth as it is in heaven. (Matthew 6:10, NIV)

So do not start worrying: "Where will my food come from? or my drink? or my clothes?" (These are the things the pagans are always concerned about.) Your Father in heaven knows that you need all these things. Instead, be concerned above everything else with the Kingdom of God and with what he requires of you, and he will provide you with all these other things. So do not worry about tomorrow; it will have enough worries of its own. There is no need to add to the troubles each day brings. (Matthew 6:31–34, GNT)

Living Fully Now and into Your Forever

What else? Make bucket lists[72] of what you want to do before you leave this life. I suggest three buckets.

I will give you a few examples to get you started.

Bucket List One: To do every day

1. Be grateful to God for every breath and my washing machine.
2. Enjoy conversation with God—and try not to do all the talking.
3. Read God's Word and even memorize what I can.
4. Love the people God puts on my path, even when that seems too hard.
5. Bring a smile with me wherever I go.

Bucket List Two: Assume you have a typical life trajectory with many years ahead.

1. See the fjords of the world I haven't seen yet (already did Alaska, British Columbia, Washington, Killary Harbour in Ireland, Somes Sound in Maine, Quebec, Scotland, Norway, and New Zealand).

---

72 John Eldredge's book, *All Things New*, teaches us to make a bucket list for our new life in the new heaven and new earth. One entry for me will be to spend 1,000 years talking with Moses. Mr. Eldredge even says we don't need to bother with these ordinary lists attached to our broken world.

2. Read all of Augustine I haven't read yet, plus Plato and St. Francis.
3. Get into God's rhythm. Norman Vincent Peale taught me that to get into God's rhythm, go into the woods away from roads, lie down on your stomach, and put your ear to the ground. You'll hear God's rhythm. I seem to be stuck on a freeway.

Bucket List Three: You suffer from a chronic disease or you have been given a limiting diagnosis. Kathleen Singh calls this enlightenment at gunpoint. This is what I call my not-much-time-left list.

1. Walk some of the world's most beautiful beaches where the sun is shining. A Sunday school teacher I had in the '70s taught me that creation is God's first Bible. Study nature and you study God.
2. Have a "Shop Hattie's Closet" event for my girlfriends and nieces. Kathi can supervise or make decisions if two want the same pair of shoes or the same necklace or the same silk blouse. I'll be there, but Kathi is nonpartial and the honest style queen. Keiko might even be able to come, which would be amazing. If Bruce has already transitioned, they can also shop the house for art that has not already been designated for someone else. Everybody knows Marilyn gets the small Kelly Mills and the Cape Cod.
3. Be where foliage is green and flowers are blooming to enjoy the metaphor of resurrection since I will soon experience it in a new way.
4. Update my Circle of Care, as I have just moved to a new town.
5. Get close to "Sister Death."

NOTE: There are five times when you want to update what you have created in these pages, especially what you include in the "My Gift to My Circle of Care" on pages 149–157. 1. Decline in health. 2. Diagnosis 3. Divorce 4. Death of someone close. 5. Every decade.

Appendices

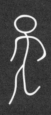

My Directive in Essay Form

HATTIE'S HEALTHCARE DIRECTIVE
Let Nature Take Its Course

When I am no longer able to do the things that are important to me such as breathe on my own, chew and swallow food, toilet myself, carry on a conversation, recognize people I know, read, etc., (unless I am healing from what is considered to be a short-term issue where full recovery is anticipated), I direct that medical care be withheld or withdrawn and that I be permitted to die naturally with only the administration of pain medications and other symptom-control medications to keep me comfortable.

Let nature take its course is my theme. When I can no longer speak for myself, my trusted proxies will execute the following:

Hospice care should be ordered by either a doctor who is on the case or accessed (a simple phone call) by a family member or either of my healthcare advocates who both have my durable power of attorney for healthcare, Falyn Curtis or Dr. Pat Gary. If I have some sort of calamity in public, I realize that 911 will be called, CPR will get done to me if needed to keep me alive and I will get taken to an ER. Hopefully, very quickly after that, my healthcare advocates will be contacted and they will implement this plan. If I have a calamity at home, do not call 911. No healthcare provider, including EMTs, is allowed to touch me without consultation with Ms. Curtis or Dr. Gary. Dr. Gary said she would not let me die on the floor, so I guess someone is allowed to pick me up off the floor and put me on a bed or sofa. Don't put me on the white sofas, as you know things can get messy.

Forbidden Treatments/Override

I forbid and choose to forego CPR, surgery, chemotherapy, dialysis, tests, ventilation, feeding tubes (no tube down my nose and no percutaneous endoscopic gastrostomy tube), blood transfusions, antibiotics or IV hydration. I do not choose to die in a hospital or any other institution. The exception would be a Hospice in-patient facility due to the need for its pain and symptom management capabilities.

I authorize the withholding of artificially provided food, intravenous fluids, and other nourishments. If I cannot give directions regarding my medical care I intend for my family and physicians to honor this declaration as the final expression of my right to refuse medical care, food and water and I accept the consequences of that refusal.

No family member—my husband, my siblings, my nieces and nephews—may override this directive and no family member is in charge of my death and dying. I am in charge per these directives even if I have lost my mind (cognitive functioning), or my ability to communicate. My advocates agree they will follow this directive.

Comfort Care ONLY

A few more details to be very clear . . .

If I cannot feed myself, swallow, enjoy food, prepare simple meals, toilet myself, walk to my mailbox, (in healthcare-speak, these are called the activities of daily living or ADL) recognize my family and friends, carry on a conversation, read, write emails, and search the Internet, I want no more doctor's offices, no more hospitals, I will stop taking any medication (except to mitigate unpleasant symptoms such as pain, nausea, shortness of breath or agitation) and will not call 911. This means DNH, do not hospitalize. It means keep me comfortable and let nature take its course.

This means, I may stop eating and drinking and do not want to be forced to eat or take water. I want hospice care with Falyn Curtis and/or Dr. Gary (who both have my durable power of attorney for healthcare) making sure that everyone sticks to this plan. This means I should die within 7–10 days if I am a textbook case, however, experience teaches and experts say that it could take longer. It could take much longer as no one of us is in control. Don't worry about this because hospice clinicians will be on the scene and you will not be alone. They have seen it all and will be a comfort to you.

If, in the dying process, I say I am changing my mind about all of this: Do not listen, and stick to this written plan. If I cannot speak for myself or if my mind—cognitive functioning—is gone, I forbid anyone to alter this directive and I repeat, do not force me to take in food or water. I have learned from palliative care nurses that feeding some people is painful to them so don't imagine that feeding me is loving me.

Feeding me is not loving me.

Not feeding me is not you killing me.

Not feeding me is letting nature takes its course.

Not feeding me is putting me fully, wholly and kindly into the hands of my God.

Please recall the words of Jesus, "He who eats me shall live by me, and shall live forever" (John 6:51). This dying process is not physical, it is not medical, it is transcendent; and comfort only comes from God bringing me to himself. Read page 199 of Dallas Willard's book *The Divine Conspiracy*, and you will understand better what I am saying.

I am ready to go back to God. I am ready to go home. You can hang up a sign that says, "SHE'S GOING HOME." Then when I die, you can flip over the sign and it should read, "SHE'S GONE HOME."

Please realize that these instructions will be followed not based upon treatments starting or stopping; these instructions will be followed based upon how I choose to live out my last days. These instructions apply even if all I have is dementia. I do not want to be given any medical treatments or food or water when I reach the point I have described at the top of this page. Only provide palliative care with the help of hospice professionals.

If Bruce is still living and he doesn't want me to die in our bed or in our house, I understand that and I suppose a hospice service has a bed for me somewhere.

Send Me off in Song

I do hope you'll come and visit if you like but never feel that you have to and don't come because you feel guilty. Only come if you want to see how it is all working and if you have something to read to me or tell me.

Please play music . . . hymns, praise and worship songs, opera arias (no Wagner and only the big famous songs, never the whole opera), all the famous symphonic works (no Mendelssohn and no Mozart, as they bore me and I love the Russians). Play Bach any time you don't know what else to play. Or, play any Yo-Yo Ma recording. No TV. Play Casting Crowns, Natalie Grant, Selah, David Phelps, Larnelle Harris. At least once a day, play my favorite song, "Give Me Jesus" performed by Fernando Ortega.

Have some fun! You can read the Psalms out loud but not the laments or the ones about being chased by enemies.

Thank you, sweet ones. I am singing in my head, "Swing Down Chariot, Come and Let Me Ride" and "Angel Band." You'll find these songs in my stack of CDs if you want to sing along.

My latest sun is sinking fast, my race is nearly run
My strongest trials now are past, my triumph is begun
I know I'm nearing holy ranks of friends and kindred dear
I brush the dew of Jordan's banks, the crossing must be near
I've almost gained my heav'nly home, my spirit loudly sings
The holy ones behold they come; I hear the noise of wings
O come, angel band come and around me stand
O bear me away on your snowy wings to my immortal home
O bear me away on your snowy wings to my immortal home

CliffsNotes[73] for the Psalms

To get ready to die—to really LIVE—to really LIVE fully into your forever—get hooked on the Psalms.

I know it's a big book. Here's a way to get you started.

Baby Boomers suffer from more depression, more alcoholism, and have more psychiatric problems than our grandparents did. While I am not telling you to drop your anti-depressant drug, if you let the Psalms sink into your bones, you will be changed. I promise that one Psalm per day can help keep the blues away.

In tribute to the way many Baby Boomers got through school, I have written these CliffsNotes[74] for the Psalms. This way, even on busy days, you can just grab a tiny dose of greatness. Do not think this is as good as reading the Psalms. It is not. Think of a song you love—let's use "Amazing Grace," since it is so famous and loved. Imagine meeting a person who has never heard that song. I could say to her, "There's this wonderful song called 'Amazing Grace,' and it is about God's love for us." From that, can she really get the power of the song? Of course not. But, it might inspire her to go find the song on YouTube and listen.

These short sentences are intended to inspire you to fall in love with the only prayers we really need, the only poetry we can feast on day in and day out. These are the prayers that will bring you to God now, right now. You don't have to wait to die; you can have all of him now; you can have heaven now.

Psalm 1: The one who meditates on God will not wither.
Psalm 2: God protects those who depend on him.
Psalm 3: God shields from trouble and delivers those who call to him.
Psalm 4: God alone keeps us safe.
Psalm 5: God welcomes the one who seeks him.
Psalm 6: Plea for God to come to the rescue.
Psalm 7: Plea for God to be fair.
Psalm 8: Praise to God, whose name echoes around the world.
Psalm 9: Praise for God's justice and plea for more.
Psalm 10: Praise for God's justice and plea for him to intervene.

Psalm 11: God is watching us all and he is righteous.
Psalm 12: God will keep the needy safe and give protection from the wicked.

---

73 About CliffsNotes, accessed December 2, 2018, https://www.cliffsnotes.com/discover-about.
74 Ibid.

Psalm 13: Plea for help and praise that God is good to those who trust him.

Psalm 14: Man is in a pitiful state, but God rescues the ones who do right.

Psalm 15: The honest, kind, generous, promise keepers will be protected by God.

Psalm 16: Plea for safety and protection and praise for God's direction.

Psalm 17: Plea for justice and protection from evil and recognition of God's power.

Psalm 18: Praise for God's direction and power.

Psalm 19: Praise for God's creation and guidance then a plea for a fresh start.

Psalm 20: God rescues and gives victory to those who love him.

Psalm 21: God destroys evil and blesses those who give him glory.

Psalm 22: Plea for help and praise to God that he always rescues.

Psalm 23: Praise to God for meeting our every need forever.

Psalm 24: Praise to God for his creation and instruction on how to reach him.

Psalm 25: God will reveal his truth to the humble, hear our confession and bless us.

Psalm 26: Those who trust God praise him, pray for mercy, and avoid evil.

Psalm 27: God is my only source; he hears my prayers so I am not afraid.

Psalm 28: God hears the prayers of those who call for help, and he strengthens them.

Psalm 29: Thanksgiving that after darkness, joy comes in the morning, over and over.

Psalm 30: Praise to God that in spite of my weakness, he saves me over and over.

Psalm 31: God rescues those who seek him and delivers justice to the evil.

Psalm 32: Command to give God glory for forgiveness and a new start.

Psalm 33: Give God praise as his power is all we need.

Psalm 34: Run to God and he will rescue you from all your fears, because he is good.

Psalm 35: Plea for help and protection from bad people and praise that God hears.

Psalm 36: Praise for God's love and the protection he gives to those who love him.

Psalm 37: Stay calm. Wait on God, for those who follow God's path win.

Psalm 38: Plea for help and confession of sin and weakness.

Psalm 39: Lord, I am pathetic and nothing but a vapor. My only hope is in you.

Psalm 40: Because I trusted God and waited for him he saved me from the slimy pit.

Psalm 41: Praise for God's healing mercies and his protection from my enemies.

Psalm 42: Even though things are very dark, I am confident God will come to my aid.

Psalm 43: Only God turns depression into praise, darkness to light, sadness to joy!

Psalm 44: All of our past victories are from God, so we ask God for more help now.

Psalm 45: Jesus Christ is King, so we must drop everything and follow only him.

Psalm 46: Praise God, because he protects us.

Psalm 47: Praise God, because he is in charge of everything.

Psalm 48: God heaps goodness on us and guides us to the end of time.

Psalm 49: Only God can save us; we cannot save ourselves.

Psalm 50: God demands my undivided attention, my praise, worship and respect.

Psalm 51: Ask for forgiveness, beg for mercy, and promise to give God praise.

Psalm 52: God gives mercy to those who ask for help.

Psalm 53: Our hope in God is our only cure from sin.

Psalm 54: A plea for help and praise for God's rescue.

Psalm 55: Give your problems to God. He'll handle them, plus wipe out your enemies.

Psalm 56: Plea for God to hold enemies at bay, and praise to God for saving me.

Psalm 57: God hides me in the shelter of his wings; I sing glory be to God my savior.

Psalm 58: Evil powers are pervasive. God wipes them out and rewards the right doers.

Psalm 59: God is our refuge and our only safe place.

Psalm 60: We are helpless without God.

Psalm 61: When I am weak, God is my solid rock and the wing I hide under.

Psalm 62: All hope, all life, all protection, all strength is from God, and we are nothing.

Psalm 63: God holds my right hand; I will not fall, and he will destroy my enemies.

Psalm 64: Fly to God and give him glory, for he is our safe place.

Psalm 65: Thanks be to God for removing the weight of our sin and for blessing us.

Psalm 66: God hears me; God saves me; God puts me on the right path.

Psalm 67: If God's people give him praise, the world will take note.

Psalm 68: God is to be praised, for he protects us from our enemies.

Psalm 69: God will rescue the humble and destroy the enemy of the godly.

Psalm 70: Plea to God that he derail my enemies and come quickly to rescue me.

Psalm 71: I have had plenty of trouble in my life, and you, God, you will restore me.

Psalm 72: Evil will be defeated; my God is in charge; the earth pulses with his glory.

Psalm 73: The struggling one finds peace with God. God himself holds my right hand.

Psalm 74: God, your reputation is on the line; save me and all will see your greatness.

Psalm 75: God rules; God delivers. He punishes the wicked and saves the righteous.

Psalm 76: God makes thing right. God deserves praise.

Psalm 77: I'm a mess, but God comes to my rescue.

Psalm 78: Men and women are pathetic and God is good. God keeps rescuing.

Psalm 79: Evil roams and seems to win and we continue to praise God who saves us.

Psalm 80: Praise for what God did to save us in the past; prayer for more rescuing.

Psalm 81: God promises that if we listen to him, he will solve all of our problems.

Psalm 82: People are sinful; only God is good; only God can be trusted.

Psalm 83: Plea to stamp out evil, and praise for God's singular power to do it.

Psalm 84: With God we have heaven here; a light to guide; a shield to protect.

Psalm 85: God can be trusted; those who look to him will find a clear path.

Psalm 86: God rescues; God protects; God listens; God restores.

Psalm 87: God is the source of every necessity and of every joy.

Psalm 88: Crying out to God is our only way to get ourselves out of trouble.

Psalm 89: God's mercy endures. God corrects and saves those who praise him.

Psalm 90: Without God's love we are nothing more than dust.

Psalm 91: Those who trust in God are protected by him and his angel army.

Psalm 92: God alone stands the test of time and he brings the faithful with him.

Psalm 93: God rules the world—the sea, the mountains, everything.

Psalm 94: Plea to God that he punish evil and praise that he saves right-doers.

Psalm 95: Praise that the God of the universe is my personal protector and guide.

Psalm 96: Sing praises to God and know that he is coming to set things right.

Psalm 97: God hates evil; he plants light and joy in the hearts of those who hate evil.

Psalm 98: Sing and play instruments in praise to our God, for he will set things right.

Psalm 99: God is in charge of everything and still hears and answers our prayer.

Psalm 100: Praise God and be thankful that he is good all of the time.

Psalm 101: I am praising you, God, for your love and justice, by trying to please you.

Psalm 102: Complaint that I am falling apart, and confidence God will rescue me.

Psalm 103: I bless God for making me right, since I am just a pitiful handful of mud.

Psalm 104: My God is great, the Creator of all; without my God every living thing dies.

Psalm 105: Sing out to the whole world that our God always rescues the faithful.

Psalm 106: We keep sinning and God keeps saving (if and when we call out for help).

Psalm 107: Our stupidity gets us into deep trouble, and thankfully God pulls us out.

Psalm 108: Plea that God slay the enemies and praise that God can.

Psalm 109: Wickedness oppresses but your goodness, God, will heal my brokenness.

Psalm 110: Be patient and trust God while he wins all the battles.

Psalm 111: Knowing, trusting, and loving God are the ways to a good life.

Psalm 112: God gives a happy, secure, generous heart to those who love him.

Psalm 113: Praise God all day, every day, because he solves every problem.

Psalm 114: God takes us away from, and through, every evil to deliver us to safety.

Psalm 115: Praise to the one true God who helps me; the little gods are useless.

Psalm 116: I love you, Lord, because you heard my cry for help. You made things right.

Psalm 117: Praise God; he is the only constant in our lives. God alone delivers 24/7.

Psalm 118: My God is bigger than any problem. He shines light on those who love him.

Psalm 119: God's Word—his teachings—are forever. It is only truth that I must seek.

Psalm 120: Take your troubles to God.

Psalm 121: God guards your every move 24/7, because he never sleeps.

Psalm 122: God expects all who trust him to live in peace.

Hattie Bryant

Psalm 123: Plea for mercy and admission that we are powerless without God.

Psalm 124: Praise to God for saving us over and over and over again.

Psalm 125: God makes those who trust him so strong they can endure any hardship.

Psalm 126: God rescued us before and he'll do it again; it seems too good to be true.

Psalm 127: We are completely dependent upon God. Anything we do alone is silly.

Psalm 128: God pours goodness on those who trust and obey him.

Psalm 129: God will destroy the evildoers and make right the righteous.

Psalm 130: I pray and wait on God. He has always saved me, he'll do it again.

Psalm 131: You are God and I am not, so I am patient and happy to rest in your arms.

Psalm 132: Praise to God for kept promises.

Psalm 133: We are blessed when we get along with each other.

Psalm 134: Those who praise God receive God's blessings.

Psalm 135: The God who made everything and controls everything holds my hand.

Psalm 136: God's love for me never stops; he never quits; he never runs out on me.

Psalm 137: Cries for help.

Psalm 138: Thanksgiving and praise that God has rescued me, and prayer for more.

Psalm 139: Praise for marvelously making me, knowing me, and loving me.

Psalm 140: Lord, you are my God. Save me from people who want to harm me.

Psalm 141: God, I am focused on you; protect me; do not let people kill me.

Psalm 142: Lord, I have never been so low and there is no one but you to help me.

Psalm 143: Lord, I am yours. I need protection. Hurry, I need it now.

Psalm 144: I praise you, God. You keep rescuing and blessing me, because I trust you.

Psalm 145: God, you shine! You are in control; you are the source of all goodness.

Psalm 146: I praise you, God, for you are in charge and you are making things right.

Psalm 147: God, you delight in all of us who trust in you; we are in awe of your power.

Psalm 148: Praise the Lord! You are the Creator of all and you pick me up when I fall.

Psalm 149: I am happy in you, Lord. I am singing your praises. You are my all in all.

Psalm 150: Praise the Lord. Let everything that has life praise the Lord.

Note: Psalm 118 is the favorite psalm of Saint Augustine and Martin Luther, so my CliffsNotes[75] could be even shorter if you just read that one psalm. However, I bet you can't read just one.

---

75 Ibid.

Cut-Out Pages to Copy and Share

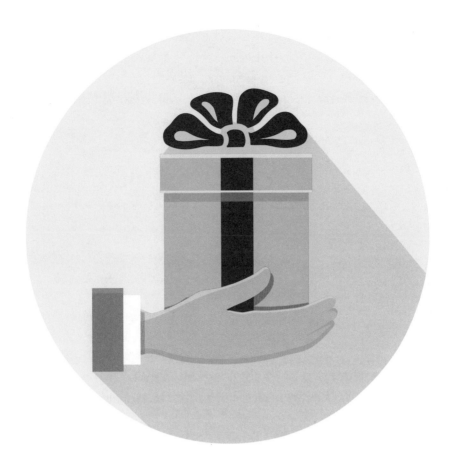

My Gift to My Circle of Care

Dear Everyone in My Circle of Care,

I have been thinking about my future, and want you to know that I hope you will be part of it. You can see from these pages that I have chosen a durable power of attorney for healthcare, also known as a proxy. You can see how I want the last few years, weeks, months, and days of my life to unfold. Please know that I am not afraid to leave this earth, as I have been thinking about being with Jesus in heaven and look forward to seeing his face. I am not afraid and I don't want you to be afraid for me or for yourself. Please honor what I have given you here.

With these instructions provided now, I pray I have lifted any burden that anyone might feel about my well-being. I want you to know that I have nothing but love in my heart for you and what you have been to me throughout the time we have been together on this earth.

My goal is that my death will be a worship experience for me and for anyone who might be present. Let me leave with the words of Jesus, "Father, I give you my life."

Our Father will reach down and bring me to himself and those around will see his grace and glory. It will be YES and AMEN.

These individuals are in my Circle of Care and will receive copies of these instructions:
1.
2.
3.
4.
5.
6.
7.
8.
9.
10.

I request that my instructions be respected. My named proxy is the person who will make sure this happens if I can no longer speak to physicians on my own behalf.

Check the statement that fits you best:

☐ It's OK with me if keeping me alive requires unlimited resources paid for by insurance (private/Medicaid/Medicare), my own savings/the savings of family, and makes heavy demands on the time and emotions of family and friends.

☐ It's OK with me if keeping me alive requires unlimited resources paid for by insurance (private/Medicaid/Medicare) and my own savings. However, I do not want my care to be a financial or emotional burden on my family. So, when my money runs out, let me go naturally. I realize that this choice means I might have nothing left to leave to my children and grandchildren.

☐ It's OK to keep me alive so long as it's paid for by insurance (private/Medicaid/Medicare). So, when my benefits run out, let me go naturally. That way I can leave any assets to my family.

☐ I am beginning to understand that keeping me alive at all costs (money and the efforts required of so many others) is not what I want for my life. I want to leave gently with people sorry to see me go rather than hoping I will go.

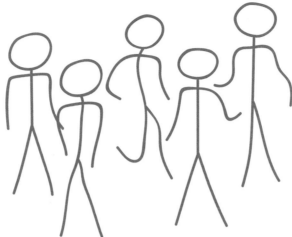

When I am frail or seriously ill, I want my family, physicians, and all of those in my Circle of Care to focus on (please circle one):

**Quantity
(number of days)**   **Quality
(the stuff of my day)**

These are the things that are important to me while I am here on this earth:

If my healthcare providers state I will never regain these functions, I am to be provided care that will keep me comfortable and pain-free until I die.

In order to live the life I desire, it is important for me to retain the ability to: (initial all that apply to you)

☐ Share my thoughts through words, gestures or assistive devices.
☐ Understand what people are saying to me.
☐ Know that I am hungry and be able to swallow.
☐ Chew and swallow food which means I do not want a feeding tube.
☐ Take care of my own toileting needs.
☐ Take a bath or shower with or without assistance.
☐ Interact in social settings.

Other functions that are important to me:

_____

_____

_____

_____

_____

If I have lost any of these functions that are important to me, do no not attempt resuscitation, please avoid calling 911, and please avoid taking me to a hospital. Please call for palliative medicine only. Keep me comfortable and let nature take its course. (Use a pen or marker to redact this, if you wish.)

For My Healthcare Proxy, Family, Friends, and Healthcare Providers

Durable Power of Attorney for Healthcare Decisions

Based upon the work you see I have done on the preceding pages,
I want you to know that if and when I can no longer speak for myself,

_____

Address: _____

_____

City/State/Zip Code: _____

Phone No: _____

will be in charge of making sure that my wishes are respected. If this person is not

available, the alternate proxy/surrogate is:

_____

Address: _____

_____

City/State/Zip Code: _____

Phone No: _____

I,_____being of sound mind,
do hereby designate the above to serve as my Attorney-in-Fact, for the purpose of
making medical treatment decisions for me (including the withholding or withdrawal
of life-sustaining procedures, nutrition, hydration) should I be diagnosed and certified
as having an irreversible condition and be comatose, incompetent, or otherwise
mentally or physically unable to make such decisions for myself.

My named proxies are strong people who know me well and need only to refer to my answers to the questions in this plan which I have written in my own hand or have dictated to a caregiver.

I understand the full import of this directive and I am emotionally and mentally competent to make this directive.

My Name (In Print): _____

My Signature: _____ Date: _____

Address: _____

In our joint presence,_____
who is of sound mind and eighteen (18) years of age, or older, voluntarily dated and signed this writing or directed it to be dated and signed for the grantor.

Witness 1 Name: _____

Address: _____

Witness Signature: _____ Date: _____

Witness 2 Name: _____

Address: _____

Witness Signature: _____ Date:_____

I have made multiple copies of these pages and have shared them with those listed above. Thanks to everyone for being part of making my dreams for a peaceful passing to Jesus easy for me and everyone involved.

"And now he has made all of this plain to us by the coming of our Savior Jesus Christ, who broke the power of death and showed us the way of everlasting life through trusting him" (2 Timothy 1:10, TLB).

MY CIRCLE OF CARE

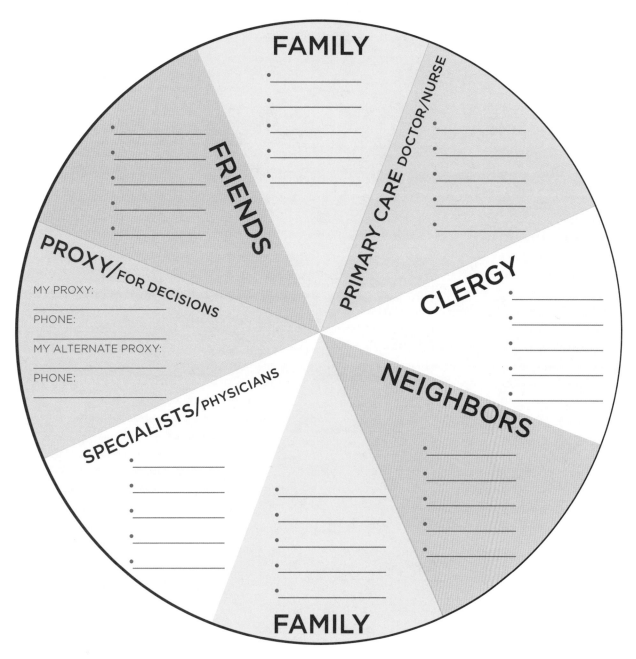

Make copies and share with all you include.